The Story of Life

The Life We All Try to Find

PAT STARK

The Story of Life
by Pat Stark
Published by Covenant Publishing House
26 Lake Wire Drive
PO Box 524
Lakeland, FL 33802-0524
www.thecovenantcenter.com

Editing by Lawrence Hughes
Project managed by Heather Celoria
Layout & Design by Tara Allen
Cover art by Krivosheev Vitaly/Shutterstock.com

Copyright © 2015 Pat Stark

All rights reserved. No part of this publication may be reproduced, stored in a retrievable system, or transmitted in any form or by any means, electronic, mechanical, photocopying, recording, or otherwise, without prior written permission of the publisher.

Printed in the United States of America

Library of Congress Control Number: 2015934760

ISBN: 0692396543
ISBN-13: 978-0-692-39654-4

Some names and details of the story have been changed, and any similarity between the names and stories of individuals described in this book to individuals known to readers is purely coincidental.

All Scriptures, unless otherwise indicated, are taken from the Holy Bible, New International Version, © 1973, 1978, 1984, by International Bible Society.

DEDICATION

This book is dedicated to all who are hungry and thirsty for more of true life. To those who desire to reclaim the life that has been stolen through the pain of this broken world, discovering the true life Jesus paid to restore. And to Jesus Christ who has patiently and faithfully walked with me all these years on my own journey of restoration and through the discovery of who I was originally created to be.

CONTENTS

	Before We Begin	i
	Introduction	vii
1	Searching for Life That Satisfies	1

Made for the Garden
Desiring More
True Life
Living with an Alive Heart: A Clue to Authentic Living

2	Reinterpreting Life	17

Confusion Between God and the Enemy
Healing Takes Place Through Facing Our Reality
The World in Which We Were Originally Created to Live
The Two Trees in the Garden of Eden
The Tree of Knowledge of Good and Evil
The Tree of Life

3	Finding God's Peace in the Struggles of Our Lives	33

The Different Seasons of Our Lives
We Live with Mixture

4	Reconciliation, Redemption, Restoration	53

The Atmosphere We Carry and the "Name" It Gives Us
The Atmosphere of a Home
Renaming
Real or Legitimate Shame
False or Illegitimate Shame and a Shame-Based Identity
Discovering God's Truth About Us

5	Grieving Our Disappointed Desires and Losses	69

Releasing Our Losses Through Grief
My Own Journey of Grief
Common Symptoms of Grief
My Letter

6	Handling Our Messy Emotions and Bringing Them Under God's Control	91
	Peace at Any Cost is Not Peace	
	Our Longings and Desires	
	Taking Back Our Story	
7	Uncovering Our Own Hearts and Discovering the Essence of Who We Really Are	111
	Our Imaginations Reclaimed	
	True Scriptural Pictures: Using Our Imaginations Well	
8	Our Cooperation with God in Becoming Who We Were Designed to Be	123
	Questions to Ask Yourself	
	Understanding the Times and Seasons of Our Lives	
	Two Winds	
	Learning to Abide	
9	Learning to Live with Peace in a World of Turmoil and Uncertainty	141
	The Bigger Picture of Our Lives	
10	Viewing Even Death from an Eternal Perspective	149
	The Fruit of Redemption	
	Living with Peace	
	Coming to Terms with Death as a Part of Life	
	"Loving Not Their Lives Even Unto Death" (Rev. 12:11)	
	The End of the Story	
	A Partial Emotions List	165

ACKNOWLEGEMENTS

Thanks to Richard & Becky Maisenbacher and The Covenant Center for helping me discover I had treasures to release and for giving me the freedom to stretch without the fear of judgment.

Many thanks to Larry for his invaluable help with the editing and excellent suggestions. I am so grateful to Heather for her editing, design, answers to numerous questions, as well as tying things up for me. Thanks to Tara for formatting and putting it all together. Thanks to Tori and Trish for their photo help – I so appreciate you. It could never have been released without you all.

Thanks to all of you who have faithfully walked with me on my personal journey of discovery and healing. Your encouragement has been a blessing. My personal restoration is ongoing and I continually learn much from each of you. A special thanks to my wonderful family. Each one of you means so much to me – more than you will ever know. A large part of my pressing through the pain of my own journey was so a way could be made for each of you to become who you were truly created to be. It is exciting to see generational curses turn into blessings!

Before We Begin...

This book has been primarily written for those who already have allowed Jesus Christ to take up residence in their lives. If you are not sure he has yet done that, but you felt drawn to pick up the book, it is most likely because the Spirit of God has been calling to you. However it is also possible that even thinking about God calling you is a foreign concept, and you are not sure whether you have a personal relationship with Jesus Christ or not. In fact the whole idea of it might seem strange, but the good news is -- you can know for certain today!

We were never meant to just struggle through life on our own because we have a loving God who was willing to part with his own Son so that Jesus could come to this earth for a very specific purpose. You! He has patiently waited and knocked very quietly on each heart's door to be invited in. His desire has always been to take up residence within our lives, so we never have to be alone again. Jesus knows first-hand just how overwhelming this life can be. He experienced it himself in a horrific way as he was having to release his own life and be hung on a cross. That one historical act makes a way of new life possible for all of us who are willing to personally receive it.

In the hours preceding the cross, the Bible describes Jesus as being "overwhelmed with anguish" to the point of blood emanating from the pores of his skin. Just in the days leading up to his crucifixion, Jesus experienced many of the same emotions we do when facing various trials in our own lives. He also felt rejected, abandoned, betrayed by those he cared about, overwhelmed, misunderstood, mocked, ridiculed, beaten, abused, and so much more. He is truly able to understand our struggles and our pain. What Jesus experienced, certainly wasn't fair as it isn't for many of us as well.

Hebrews 12:2 tells us that Jesus willingly went through all that plus death by a horrific form of punishment in order to save us from the consequences of a choice recorded in Genesis chapter three. The decision of Adam and Eve to be their own god, by rejecting their Creator and doing things their own way, changed the course of history on this earth forever. In order to reverse the horrific results of their choice, it was necessary for Jesus to enter the pain of our separation from God and become one with us in our humanity. He took our sin and man's punishment for that decision upon himself. Now we could be totally forgiven for the sin of choosing to be our own god by doing things ourselves in our own way. The Bible describes the willfulness of mankind in this way: *"We all, like sheep, have gone astray, each one of us has turned to his own way; and the Lord laid on him the iniquity of us all."* (Isaiah 53:6)

In his wonderful devotional, My Utmost For His Highest, Oswald Chambers wrote: *"The disposition of sin is not immorality and wrong-doing, but the disposition of self-realization – I am my own god."*

When we receive the sacrifice Jesus made and invite him into our lives, he takes up residence *in us* and makes an *exchange with us*. The exchange Jesus makes is that he takes our sin, rejection, and shame upon himself and instead gives us his acceptance, forgiveness, and righteousness. We sure get the good end of the bargain!

Our part: To receive him (John 1:12-13). *"Yet to all who received him, to those who believed in his name, he gave the right to become children of God – children born not of natural descent, nor of human decision or a husband's will, but born of God."*

Exchange: (2 Corinthians 5:21) *"God made him who had no sin to be sin for us so that in him we might become the righteousness of God."*

The new life he offers us is a free gift; we don't deserve it, haven't earned it and because he paid for it, we don't have to. But, we have to receive his gift and give him our will in exchange for his. No matter how much of a mess we might be, he desires to take up residence within us and walk with us through our trials, our pain, our struggle, our messes. His desire, revealed in Isaiah 61:2, is to – *"bestow on them a crown of beauty instead of ashes..."*. Many of us have found ourselves buried in ashes – just a plain mess that we haven't known how to get out of.

"For it is by grace you have been saved through faith – and this not from yourselves, it is the gift of God – " (Ephesians 2:8). We have nothing to do but receive that free gift of salvation and new life through Jesus Christ. It's as if Jesus is standing before you with his arms outstretched offering you an extremely valuable, beautifully gift-wrapped package that is totally unearned and undeserved. All you have to do is receive it! Will you join with so many of us who have received that gift and pray the prayer at the end?

When we are willing to receive the gift of eternal life that cost him *his* life, many blessings come along with it. We receive an assurance of salvation that as we pass from this life to the next, we will be welcomed eternally into the presence of God. There is no longer any doubt as to what will happen to us when we die. But that is just one of the many aspects of peace we receive. Jesus is like a beautiful diamond with many facets that sparkle with life.

We also then have someone who desires to stick closer than a brother as we walk through the struggles, joys, and hardships of this life. We no longer have to feel alone trying to survive and just figure things out on our own. A process is begun of learning how to walk with Jesus moment by moment in the uncertainties of life in this broken world.

The Spirit of Jesus (the Holy Spirit) begins to change our hearts from the inside out. We enter a journey of life, discovering what real living was meant to look like, and the purposes for which we were created. But all of these changes in us come through an ongoing surrendering of our wills and a willingness to allow him to continue to lead us. Once we get the right starting place for our journey, we can joyfully cooperate in uncovering who we really are, and what our life was originally meant to be about. The joy of it all is the discovery that true life really fits us!

"Jesus answered, 'I am the way and the truth and the life. No one comes to the Father except through me." (John 14:6)

Are you weary of just getting by? Then listen to the words of Jesus in Matthew 11:28-30, *"Come to me, all of you who are weary and burdened, and I will give you rest. Take my yoke upon you and learn from me, for I am gentle and humble in heart, and you will find rest for your souls. For my yoke is easy and my burden is light."* When we try to go it alone it is weary, but as we learn how to be yoked with Jesus, just as two oxen are in one yoke together, walking in harmony and unison, the burden becomes light. He is calling to you, can you hear him? Will you say, "yes"?

Father God, thank you for sending your son, Jesus to this earth to experience the difficulties of life just as I do, and then thank you, Jesus, for being willing to go all the way through the horrific abuse and beatings to die on a cross for me personally. Thank you that you saw me as, "a pearl of great price" that was worth the giving up of your life! As I confess to you my demands of wanting my own way, I give my life, my sinful nature, and all the guilt I have carried to you. Thank you that you know that we have all messed up and come short, but you are still faithful to forgive all my sins and cleanse me from all my unrighteousness. (Romans 3:23,24 & 1 John 1:9).

Jesus, I come to you now and invite you to come into my life to walk with me on this new path of living. Thank you that I am truly born again! (John 3:5-8) *Thank you that I now know I will spend eternity with you.*

Please give me a new heart and a new way of living – (Ezekiel 36:26) *I am weary of the way that seemed like life to me, but really only brought "death".* (Proverbs 16:25)

Thank you that now, when my life on this earth is finished, I will see you face to face with a joyful, "Welcome home, my good and faithful servant. Come, take the place I have prepared for you from the foundation of the world."

"I tell you the truth, whoever hears my word and believes him who sent me has eternal life and will not be condemned; he has crossed over from death to life." (John 5:24)

Introduction

Almost two years ago in 2013, I felt the Spirit of God asking me to write a book with him entitled, The Story of Life. However, except for a few paragraphs to put in my iPad, nothing much was coming forth from within me to actually write down. Having learned a long time ago that anything I have of value to give to others must first be experienced as broken bread that gives life to me, I never write anything until it comes from my heart. Since nothing further seemed to be flowing, even though I was obedient to write down what little I had, I then closed the file for a year.

At the beginning of the summer of 2014, I felt an anointing rising within me to return to it, and then the flow began. With it was an urgency to complete this book over the summer even though I had very little actual time to devote to it. Nevertheless, I tried to be obedient with small snatches of time here and there. Every time I did that, the flow would begin again. Then a prophetic word came forth regarding the creative arts, and that this was the time to write because it was a season of anointing and release. With that confirmation, I knew that whatever else might or might not happen with this book after I wrote it, my orders were to be faithful to follow through with my part.

Why The Story of Life? As I daily meet with Christians in uncovering the hurts from their pasts that are sabotaging their lives and their peaceful, well-being, I find myself reinterpreting life to them over and over. Without our awareness, we have often very subtly, picked up fragments of the world's view of life that has tainted our thinking. Various beliefs such as, "*Life should be fair*", "*I should be happy*", "*I deserve...*" all deceive us with the lie that says, "*It's about me*". I have found most Christians unaware of that lie's influence, but nevertheless, it has too often skewed our thinking. This hidden lie has resulted in numerous unrealistic expectations and disappointments that have created the striving, anger, anxiety, and need for control plaguing us. We all long for joy and peace. The good news is -- it's available to us as we learn to live our lives from God's bigger story. For far too many, viewing the bigger picture of life from a Biblical perspective sadly seems to have gotten lost, confused, or was never understood to begin with. I was a Christian for over 25 years before I became able to see life from God's perspective instead of from my own neediness.

I have also found that numerous, earnest Christians have many bits and pieces of scripture, but those fragments too often don't seem to fit together in the cohesive story God is telling. As a result there is no clear understanding of *how* to co-labor with God in the nitty-gritty struggles that are faced by all of us every day. As I began to understand my life from a Biblical perspective, everything made sense, but it took my recognizing how much I was still trying to do life *my way* before I could cooperate!

In far too many of us, a sense of injustice and entitlement continually gets fed by the enemy of our souls who will destroy our peace in any way he can. That can create within us a quiet demand for fairness and justice here and now, and cause us to begin then to look at the future with a growing sense of unrest. I have found many Christians silently angry at God without their realizing it, for he seemingly is not cooperating with our particular needs and agendas. It's a delight for me to watch many of the people I have met with discover joy as they begin to see how those various fragments of scripture fit together into a beautiful story of real life in which their smaller story, containing even the hurts and disappointments, have a valuable part.

For me, this journey of real life began back in the year 1990. At that time I had been what I considered a serious Christian for over 25 years. I certainly loved Jesus and had put much effort into Bible learning, healing emotionally from past hurts, and generally living the Christian life, as well as ministering to others. It's interesting though how we can be truly committed to him yet still have locked closets within us that have never been opened. As a result, those parts of us have never been surrendered to him for we can only surrender that which we know. However God knew my heart and the deep cry within me to be free. He answered my prayer through the many painful circumstances he allowed that year, causing me to realize for the first time, that I was unable to hold anything together. I finally recognized that I was unable to control life or make it work out the way I thought it needed to be.

With that realization, the world I had tried to build literally fell apart, or at least it felt that way. Actually, what did fall apart was the world I had been desperately trying to create and control. And, like Humpty Dumpty, I was unable to put it back together again! It was at that point I realized I had no clue about how to do life and it was all truly too big for me! Prayer didn't seem to work the way I needed it to and the promises of the Bible seemed afar off. However, in the midst of my desperation, God arranged for me to attend a seminar that gave a Biblical view of life that changed my whole understanding of Christianity by about ten degrees. That was the beginning of my own life-altering personal discovery and what much of this book is about. It also includes many of the nuggets I presently share with those I counsel and disciple.

Why did you pick up this book? Perhaps it's because you know me and you are curious, or maybe the title intrigued you, or someone recommended it, or you could be just searching for more of what you thought life promised. Somewhere deep inside you might not be satisfied. You want more... Perhaps you are looking to gain understanding of all the random circumstances that are happening to you and in the world around you – things that make no sense and confusingly don't fit the "picture of life" you were led to believe. Maybe if you are to be very honest, you feel

Christianity as you've known it is just not working for you or perhaps you are vaguely dissatisfied with your life as it is. Somewhere buried within is a hunger for more of life than you are currently experiencing. Jesus called those who are hungry – blessed.

Is life just meant to be a series of random happenings that we have to get through as successfully as we can, and then we die? Or is it a story – our story, but even more – God's story, the one he is telling through our particular lives? If that is true, then are we actually participating in the story or are we just existing day to day trying to stay on top, keeping our heads above water? Some, doing more than existing, are consciously or even unconsciously trying to be top dog to prove, if only to themselves, that they are successful at this thing called life, that they have what it takes. It is said that even if you win the rat race you're still a rat! Is it worth it? Many who have gotten to the top have found it to be incredibly empty and not satisfying at all. A young man I know who put his all into being successful; reading all the right books, attending the best business seminars, receiving excellent mentoring, told me recently that he is beginning to discover, though it was all good, it was the wrong journey to real life.

If we make the choice to settle, to just exist, we can still feel empty, and the insatiable desire to fill our lives remains lurking under the surface. We struggle with a need to fill the emptiness with whatever seems to satisfy at the moment, whether work, pleasure, ministry, busyness, exercise, hobbies, sports, shopping, the latest food or fashions, toys, travel, the internet – stuff. And yet that quiet, gnawing ache seems impossible to satisfy for long; it is an insatiable need, almost like a bucket with a hole in it.

Join me on a journey for abundant life, a life full of grace and peace, meaning and purpose – your true life, the one you were designed for and that can only be lived from your heart.

That is life that is really life with fulfillment and joy right in the midst of a broken world! And if while you are reading, you find God's Spirit highlighting areas within your own heart that have yet to be healed, I recommend you get a copy of an earlier book I have written called, Born to Fly. It is available on Amazon in both paperback and Kindle and can help to facilitate the healing process.

My prayer for you as you read this book is from Ephesians 3:18, "*That the eyes of your heart may be enlightened in order that you may know the hope to which he has called you, the riches of his glorious inheritance in the saints*". I pray you read this book with your heart and not just from your mind alone.

CHAPTER 1
Searching for Life That Satisfies

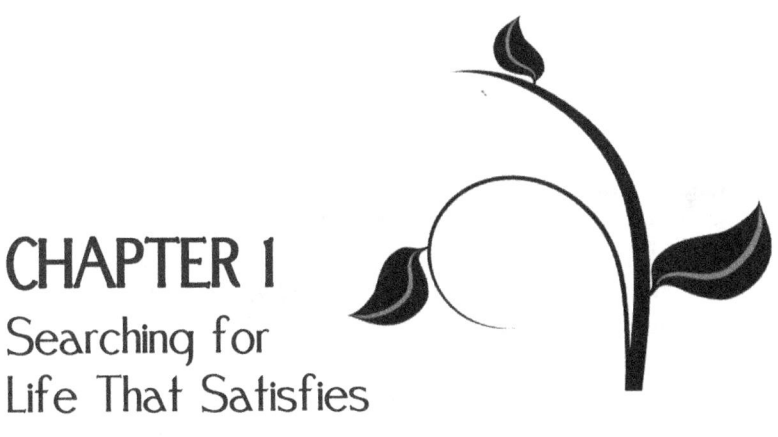

The vague sensing that we were created for more doesn't often break in for many of us until there is a forced quietness like an illness, a job loss, or being laid up for some reason. Perhaps it might even break through during a quiet, reflective time at the beach or in the mountains. Far too often, when unsettling thoughts like that begin to enter, we just find another way to be busy. That sensing however, is coming up from the truest part of us. We were designed for more and that is the reason we can become so easily dissatisfied even in the good moments and pleasures of life.

Made for The Garden

I invite you to take a walk with me back through the Garden of Eden. Far too often we read Genesis chapters one and two in a very cursory manner without taking the time to look and listen beneath the words on a page. What was life originally meant to look like? We need to know because that is the life we were made for. The ache for that life is still locked up deeply within our hearts. If we are ever to really know ourselves and what our lives are truly about, we have to see larger and struggle more deeply than most of us have been willing to do. We must wrap our arms around God's original

CHAPTER 1

design because the longings for that life still remain buried within. Even though because of the Fall, we will never be completely satisfied and full on this earth, there is great delight to be found in our co-laboring with God according to our unique design in the larger story he is telling in the earth.

"God saw all that he had made and it was very good ..." (Genesis 1:31)

"Thus the heavens and the earth were completed in all their vast array." (Genesis 2:1)

Join me in rediscovering God's beautiful creation, the one we were originally made to experience. Picture a place of such lavish beauty that has nothing to spoil it -- no weeds, thorns, thistles, crabgrass, nasty insects that destroy. Smell the fragrance of the lush and gorgeous flowers that are continually in abundant bloom. Feel the atmosphere that is crisp and clean with no heaviness or humidity, and allow the gentle breezes that refresh to brush over your face. See the animals of all kinds frolicking together without devouring one another -- the lion laying down with the lamb. There was no fear in that Garden, no anger or anguish. It was a place of peace and tranquility, of love and acceptance.

See Adam and Eve as they came fully alive with the breath of God that was blown into the clay from which they were formed. Notice their respectful caring and consideration for each other, never using each other to meet their own selfish needs, no contempt, or abuse. There was no tension, stress, or unending list of "to do's", but instead, laughter, playfulness, and joy unspeakable and full of glory. Why? The glory of God filled the Garden, the God of light himself covered them. Psalm 104:2 describes God's glory as light that he wrapped himself with as a garment. That is what they were covered with and as a result, they were naked but not ashamed (Genesis 2:25). There was no fear of failure or exposure lurking. But the best part of all -- the awesome creator God walked with them, talked, and fellowshipped with them in the cool of the day (Genesis 3:8). And then because they were created for purpose, the Lord put them in the Garden to lovingly *tend* it. Not toiling in it because that curse of toiling or stressing came in later through the Fall of man (Genesis 3:17-19); instead, fulfilling garden tending!

Notice there were two trees in midst of the Garden, one teeming with Life, and then the other that was also very appealing, the Tree of the Knowledge of Good and Evil. Genesis 2:9 describes the Garden as being full of trees of all kinds and varieties that were *"pleasing to the eye and good for food".* It wasn't as if man was deprived in any way by God's request to freely eat from any tree except from that one, the Tree of the Knowledge of Good and Evil. They had an overabundance from which to choose.

He emphatically told them if they ate of that one tree, they would *"surely die."* And die man did, not just physically at the end of a lifespan, but a part of us, deep within, died as well. Jesus came to redeem and restore us back to that original intent. No, we won't fully live the life of the Garden again until we live with God face to face in the new heaven and the new earth (Revelation 21 & 22) for Romans 8 reminds us that all of creation has now been subjected to decay. But after his resurrection, Jesus breathed the breath of life back into his disciples (John 20:21-22). It was a picture of the personal restoration we were meant to discover, not only in our spirits, but also as a flow of the life of Jesus *in us* that brings with it our purpose and destiny. Eternal life is meant to be more than going to heaven when we die as amazingly wonderful as that is. Jesus said eternal life begins when we come to know him, but we must seek and participate in that life. (John 17:3)

Tending is delightful, it's what we were personally created to do and through that we get to uniquely participate with God in the wonderful ongoing creativity he has put within each of us. But notice something very important here! They didn't begin with the *doing*, they began with the *being*. We don't get our identity from what we *do*, but from who we *"be" (are)*. Genesis 2:7 says, "*The Lord God formed the man from the dust (clay) of the ground and breathed into his nostrils the breath of life, and the man became a living being.*" Then several verses later we read in verse 15, "*The Lord God took the man and put him in the Garden of Eden to work it and take care of it.*".

Our *doing* is always meant to come out of our *being* and it's only when we discover our true *being* that is hidden deep within us that we begin to *do* in the way we were uniquely created to function. That *doing* though, is always only in cooperating with the life of Jesus within us. It is a "we", no longer an "I". *"I have been crucified with Christ and I no longer live, but Christ lives in me. The life I live in the body, I live by faith in the Son of God, who loved me and gave himself for me"* (Galatians 2:20) None of that comes easily for any of us because our natural man still struggles with the independent spirit we inherited from our forefathers. We must actually *pursue* the life we were created to live. (Psalm 139)

"*He who believes in Me--who cleaves to and trusts in and relies on Me – as the Scripture has said, out from his innermost being springs and rivers of living water shall flow (continuously).*" (John 7:38 Amplified) Anything other than that life coming from the deepest place within us, where the invited Spirit of Jesus dwells, is empty *toiling* no matter how much success we might derive from it.

Desiring More

Whether aware of it or not, most are on a search for more, something we might not even be able to describe. On a deep level of the heart, we want more than we are currently experiencing and, far too often, that indescribable desire is coming from an undefined and unexplored emptiness within. What is it that would fill that hole? Would it look like success, a certain relationship, fulfillment, satisfaction, approval, belonging, peace, joy? Not everyone would put the same words to it and you might have your own. Why are addictions of all kinds, even the seemingly acceptable ones, like food, work, exercise, fishing, or sports so consuming? Why are so many Christians addicted, even to the internet, and desperately searching for satisfaction, contentment, or peace? There's nothing wrong with the above things, but when they become hiding places from our emptiness and escapes from our internal struggles, they begin to take over little by little. Eventually, not much else of real significance begins to matter.

Just yesterday, I counseled with a couple who was using seemingly good things like work and a passion for football to escape their relational conflict. How much easier to avoid through pleasure than to face how disappointed they really were with their marriage. They went into marriage with such high hopes that were full of passion and romance, but now they felt disillusioned and disappointed in each other. Like many of us, they entered marriage with a picture of what it would look and feel like, but very little of it met their expectations. Instead of facing their relational struggle head on to discover the under-lying reasons, it was easier to just bury their disappointed desires in things that were much more pleasurable, less messy, and more manageable.

We are made for relationship because the Trinity is relational to the core and we are created in God's image and likeness. Because of that, the enemy has sought to steal, kill, and destroy us in the area of our relationships – or at the very least, get us to ignore the real issues and hide our hearts in other things that seem far less complicated. Both our own hearts and the hearts of others must be *pursued*; real relationship, even with ourselves, unfortunately doesn't just happen. However, before we can truly pursue the heart of another, we must find our own from where it has been buried under layers of hurt and our own survival system of self-protection. The opposite of love is not hate, but self-protection – to survive, we will do anything we have to in order to keep our hearts from experiencing further pain. And too often, our desperate need to survive doesn't really take into account who we hurt in the process! To discover real heart-connected relationship with others requires the willingness to begin journeying back with the Spirit of God through our own hurts in order to heal. We must then forgive and release the past in order to find our own true hearts from where they had been trampled and buried. We can only give to others what we have gotten for ourselves!

True Life

So what is true life about? And what about heart-connected, alive relationships, how do we have them? Are you willing to explore? Is life really just about achieving success, wealth, fame, fun, popularity? Is it having a great ministry; someone others gather around? Is it finding that right "someone" or losing ourselves in a family or career? Is it the American Dream? The book of Ecclesiastes tells us Solomon had it all, and yet nothing satisfied.

We have searched for real life in so many ways and through countless things, sometimes different things for different people. Many have given up their search almost completely and just tried to settle. What have you used to find your place in life and discover satisfaction and contentment? Have you used a special relationship, family, career, success? Or perhaps even a number of relationships that you have enjoyed, but somehow they never seemed to deeply satisfy – at least for very long. I'm not happy to say that years ago I discovered I had a "people addiction", desperately trying to collect people to fill the ache of loneliness left from my childhood.

How many in our society have jumped from one relationship or even one marriage to another to try to find that excitement or belonging, acceptance, peace, and joy. It has become quite common for people to go through numerous marriages or to continually reinvent themselves through the change of careers. In the end, the families from those marriages become more and more complicated and the continual career reinventions often require more education that simply increases the pile of debt and struggle. Sometimes the reinvention can be a wonderful thing of a person actually discovering their true passion, but far too often people are searching for themselves from the wrong starting place. To get to the right ending place we have to have the right beginning, otherwise we might end up in the general direction, but still miss our actual destination.

Purposefully living our lives from the inside out, walking in harmony with Jesus and discovering the way he originally designed us can bring great fulfillment and joy. However it's a journey we must be willing to take *with him* in order to truly discover our own hearts. It doesn't just come naturally, and it is opposed by the enemy of our souls, so it is something we must be willing to fight for. Too many just fight other people or the circumstances they feel are holding them back. Others beat themselves up or simply settle for life that is not really life at all. Our anger is needed to fight *for* the life the enemy has robbed. God *hates robbery*, Isaiah 61 reminds us.

One Christian I know had a good education with a lucrative career, but because of the vague dissatisfaction coming from within her, she returned to school several times. Each time Toni would take up a new major only to realize after several semesters, it wasn't satisfying her. Unfortunately though, the amount of debt she was incurring was mounting. It went on and on until Toni finally began to recognize her discontentment was coming from inside her and had little to do with a career.

CHAPTER 1

How many women have used their own children to find their identity and worth? They find their value in their child's performance whether it be in school, sports, or whatever. That is the *use* of another person, not releasing love. It can all look good on the outside, but yet harm the child, and still leave the parent feeling vaguely empty on the inside if not downright angry when the child doesn't perform to their expectation. We too often try to *pull* life from someone else to fill ourselves, cover our own shame, and satisfy the emptiness we feel within. Doing that feels to the other like they are being *consumed* or *used* instead of loved, with the frequent result that the other person desires to flee! Using another to fill ourselves is co-dependency and not Biblical love. Co-dependency uses and takes, but love honors, respects, and gives. No one is meant to be used by another – that is slavery! For relationships to be healthy, both *boundaries* and a *voice* (spoken with kindness though) are necessary. We must be free to be able to say no as well as say yes, as Jesus said.

Some of us might have searched for satisfaction and fulfillment through service or ministry. I realize that I used ministry for a number of my early years to find my own worth and belonging. I didn't ever fit with the world, and because I love Jesus, I love the Bible, and I love imparting life to people, it fit me well. I became a care-*taker* of people and their feelings that eventually burned me out (false responsibility), instead of co-laboring with Jesus in care-*giving* to others with his strength and direction. Our own *human* compassion for people will burn us out. Jesus was described as one with great compassion over and over in scripture, yet he never just *fixed* people. He was willing to allow them to hurt if that would help them heal and be freed beyond the moment. We have to be willing to love the person in the long term rather than to just *fix them* in the short term. We must be willing to love the person more than just our relationship with them. Loving them well often involves allowing them to feel emotions and consequences they might be trying to escape.

"For he wounds, but he also binds up; he injures, but his hands also heal." (Job 5:18)

Without my realizing, I was using people to fill me and give me worth instead of seeing them for themselves, and along with Jesus, loving them well. How sad. I share this, never for us to feel guilty, but so we become aware of how much we need Jesus to do an ongoing work of healing in our hearts. It's nice to see we need help, but what do we do about it? That is one of the purposes of this book because there are specific keys that unlock doors within our hearts that can bring us into a greater measure of the fullness of life we were created to live. The life Jesus paid the price to return to us.

We tend to forget we were originally created for the Garden, and deep within our human heart is still a yearning for that beautiful, perfect place of ultimate fairness and joy. We are made for so much more than the mundane. If we don't just cover it over with dullness or busyness, somewhere deep inside we become slightly aware of a hunger, a buried desire for more. We get glimpses of how life was meant to be, but then they fade because this is no longer that Garden of perfection. One day, as we are reminded in scripture, there will be that new heaven and new earth and we will finally experience that for which we were created in all its fullness. But for now, as we learn to live from our hearts in a far greater measure than we have before, we get a wonderful foretaste of what real life was meant to be.

Too often we have learned how to ignore the silent ache within our hearts by each finding our own way to cover it – sometimes with good and acceptable things, sometimes not. However, if we're honest, nothing seems to fully satisfy us. Romans chapter 8 addresses this dilemma by reminding us that as long as we live in this broken world, we will live with

CHAPTER 1

an ache, a groaning while we await the fullness that is coming in the new heaven and the new earth. But at the same time, we quietly think, "There must be more now" and there is! However uncovering that *more* involves taking a journey for the rediscovery of our own disappointed and broken hearts.

We are too often people with mixed motives, thinking our hearts are pure, but without the awareness of having buried motivations. *"Half of the wood he burns in the fire; over it he prepares his meal, he roasts his meat and eats his fill. He also warms himself...From the rest he makes a god his idol, he bows down to it and worships..."* (Isaiah 44:16-17). As Isaiah reveals, we often use things for their intended use, but then also use them to get our value and worth. Just like with the example of my own ministering years ago – I was doing a good thing in helping people, but I was also using the good thing to get personal worth and identity. That can be true of almost anything we do without even realizing it.

Like Adam and Eve, when faced with the temptation to take matters into their own hands at the Fall, we far too often are also unwilling to trust God to meet our own deepest needs and desires. We sometimes trusted more readily early on, but because of the many disappointments and betrayals, we learned it wasn't safe. Although we were born with the seeds of that mistrust and unbelief from our original parents, Adam and Eve, the lies we accepted have been reinforced within us over and over. They came in through key people in our lives that have rejected us and betrayed our trust.

This is not about blaming anyone, including ourselves, but sadly about recognizing that out of our brokenness of heart, we have often hurt ourselves and others without ever consciously meaning to do so. Without a way out, we are trapped. Because of that dilemma, deep healing of the heart is often necessary if we are to live freely with deep satisfaction and be able to love the way we were originally intended. The good news is that those are the prison doors

Jesus came to open when we are willing to join him on the journey for our true hearts.

When we allow God to reveal to us some of our mixed heart motivations, there is no condemnation, only forgiveness and a chance for further healing, growth, and contentment. God longs to give us the gift of facing ourselves and our buried desires and desperation, and then he offers us the opportunity to accept his invitation to meet him at the cross in order to make an exchange. He offers his forgiveness, and then calls to us to walk with him into a whole new way of living from the inside out, instead of trying to find our lives from the outside in. Most people look to get life from outside themselves rather than from within where Jesus dwells. They look to key people, a career, or special circumstances and happenings to satisfy, but that satisfaction is never permanent. When we look to people to fill the emptiness within us, we give them the power over us instead of God.

It is unfortunately a process, not an overnight fix. It's a process I am still involved in by listening to him daily and little by little dying to my own willfulness and the silently, demanding ways I didn't even know I had. But before I could even do that, I had to be willing to the face the hurts and buried emotions that kept me captive to a survival way of living. Now as I continue to surrender to his ways and learn to draw my life from him, I am amazed at the life he is opening up for me to join with him in living. And all this happening in my latter days – so it's never too late! At 75 plus years old, I feel in many ways, my life is just beginning with new opportunities and favor.

The way I tried to escape through ministry might be foreign to you, but you might have tried to fill yourself and escape through play or pleasure, relationships or career, and as long as you were able to dull the ache for something more, you could remain unaware that it was never enough. Others have given up on life even while they live. They have killed their desire for meaning and purpose and have lost themselves with endless hours of TV or computer games. The question must be faced that is often avoided – are you satisfied? If you were truly satisfied, you wouldn't still be reading this book!

Maybe you have not even been aware of that ache inside, but have only felt driven to keep going faster and faster. But to where and for what? To satisfy something you haven't stopped long enough to listen to or define? As long as the frantic pace of a busy life continues, we tell ourselves we don't have time to think about anything more than what we have to do tomorrow. Life is busy and full, or so we try to convince ourselves and any others around us who will listen. And then...we lose a job, get an illness, or our spouse confronts us with the desire for divorce. What happened? Too late, we sadly begin to see we were absent even though we were present and a deeper reality of life finally begins to break in.

Living with an Alive Heart: A Clue to Authentic Living

If we are to learn to live from our hearts, we have to have a better understanding of what the heart is. According to scripture it is: "*The innermost center... the reservoir of the entire lifepower. It is the center of the rational-spiritual nature of man and the seat of love and of hatred. The heart is the center of thought and conception; the heart knows. It understands, it deliberates, it reflects, and estimates.*"

"*It is the center of our feelings and affections: of joy, of pain, all degrees of ill will, of dissatisfaction, from anxiety to despair; all degrees of fear, from reverential trembling to blank terror. It is the center of moral life and the place of issue of all that is good and evil in thoughts, words, and deeds. It is where God's natural law is written in us as well as the law of grace. It is the seat of the conscience and the dwelling place of Christ in us. So it is the center of the entire man."* (Excerpts taken from Unger's Bible Dictionary)

It has been said that those who learn to draw their life from the center of their being stand at the gateway of powerful living. I have found that to be amazingly true in my own life as I am learning to live more and more from the center of my being where Jesus dwells! However, it has been necessary for me to first work with God's Spirit to recognize the shame lies that formerly occupied my center in order for that life to be released. You can't put truth on top of a lie and expect it to remain!

When we have learned to no longer fully live from our hearts due to the hurt and emotional pain we've experienced, and instead have built walls of self-protection around them, we begin to live from our minds. Our thoughts and feelings begin to get mixed-up. We sadly then can disconnect for the most part from the deepest part of us, even though our emotions often leak out inappropriately! Our bodies, minds, and hearts are meant to flow in harmony led by God's Spirit of truth. However, as you can see from the above, if we have denied a large portion of ourselves, we are no longer able to live from the deepest part of our being. Many false beliefs form in our hearts due to the hurts of the past and they can drive us, often even without our knowing where that behavior is coming from. We are then unable to make good choices even though that might be our desire. Some might put a lid on themselves morally, but are really not free. In many cases, that only contributes to living with a religious spirit.

So if the heart is the whole of our being including all of the different parts, the deepest, inner parts, and the center of our being where Jesus dwells, it is vitally important to keep it alive! The Bible says we are to guard it above all else so we don't lose it. If we are to flow from the Spirit of Jesus within us and live the life we were created to live, we must learn to work with God's Spirit in allowing the integration of all the

CHAPTER 1

different parts of us into one whole. Because of the past hurts, we have learned to compartmentalize and deny the pain, causing a separation inside. Psalm 86:11 reminds us that God desires we have an undivided heart. All true life comes from the heart. It's with the heart we believe. From our heart beliefs, both good or bad come our actions, Jesus said.

Many years ago, after discovering my own heart, I began urging my husband to find his so we could connect on a deeper level. He would become incredibly frustrated with me and say, "My heart! What are you talking about? How do I live from my heart? What does that mean anyway?" I have since realized that for many, it can be a difficult concept to grasp because we have become so accustomed to living from our intellect alone. It feels much safer to live from our minds because then we feel more in control, and living from the heart can be far too vulnerable. The truth is, however, it is risky, and even dangerous unless we have developed healthy boundaries so it is not trampled upon. Any journey to find our hearts must also include understanding personal boundaries. I describe them as a picket fence around our lives with a gate. You are in control of the gate. If someone is willing to come into your presence with respect, care, consideration, they are welcome. However, if they begin to throw their garbage around your yard, put you down, use, or abuse you, there is the right to close your gate until they can come in with respect. If we do not have healthy boundaries, we will often build walls around our hearts that are like fortresses that lock others out, or the opposite, we will find ourselves being used over and over. I highly recommend the book, <u>Boundaries</u>, by Dr. Henry Cloud and Dr. John Townsend if you are unfamiliar with the concept and necessity of personal boundaries.

I have found many husbands are clueless as to why their wives would "suddenly" have an affair or seek a divorce. As long as they were providing, they were doing their job – or so they thought. And how many wives have lost themselves in their job or children while their husbands were struggling more and more with temptation and the desire for someone, anyone, to see them. How many give their hands of loving service to their families, but never connect with their hearts. If our heart has been wounded through rejection or hurt, it has been shut down and we have learned to live life from the outside of our heart. I didn't have my heart to give for many years and didn't even know it! It's impossible to have real deep connection with another person if our heart has been closed off because unfortunately, we can't give what we don't have. This book contains a journey to search for your true heart, the one Jesus longs for you to discover and delight in with him.

CHAPTER 2
Reinterpreting Life

So what were we made for? What is the real story of life? As Christians, we know it begins for us when we walk through the door of salvation by accepting Jesus and his sacrifice for us into our lives. We know it includes the forgiveness of sin. We know we need the release of the Holy Spirit in and through us, with many referring to that as the Baptism of the Holy Spirit, and yes, we know we need his gifts operating through us. But many earnest Christians stop there while trying diligently to live the Christian lifestyle.

Could all of that just be the beginning – the doorway into real life? If you were to come to visit me, you could stand in the doorway and we could have a casual conversation or you could come inside and be a part of the fellowship and function of my home. My desire would be that you enter all the way in so we could fellowship together on a deeper heart level and really get to know one another.

Could real life be more than just survival through a series of happenings, finding a measure of success, trying to be a good honest person in the family and with others, going to church, and occasionally sharing the gospel when the opportunity arises? Or does your individual life matter and have a larger purpose? In order to discover that, we need to go back to the

CHAPTER 2

larger story that God has been telling throughout the history of man.

Confusion Between God and the Enemy

I meet with a number of Christians every week to help them with emotional healing and discipling needs. Too often when a person first comes to see me, it doesn't take long to discover they have had God mixed up with Satan who is the enemy of their souls, in some very subtle ways. Satan is the thief who has tried to steal, kill, and destroy them; he is the accuser who accuses day and night according to the scriptures. In some cases, part of the angst and struggle that brought them to me in the first place was connected to this confusion. Some common questions are, "*Why did God allow such and such to happen to me?*" It might have been something that happened in early childhood, or perhaps, even last week to them or to someone they loved.

The scenario goes something like this: "*He could have prevented it – he's God!*" "*Why didn't he stop it or intervene in my circumstance? He took care of others!*" "*Why did he give me those parents who weren't really there for me?*" "*If he's the provider, why didn't he provide, and now look, I'm losing my house!*" "*Why doesn't he change my husband, my wife, my child, I've prayed faithfully?*" "*I've prayed and prayed for healing and I'm getting worse!*" "*Why does one thing after another keep happening to me – I feel I'm cursed!*" "*Why did he allow me to be abused?*" "*Where was he then?*" "*How does he expect me to really trust him?*" "*He didn't care, why should I?*" "*I love him, but I can't trust him!*" "*It's not fair!*"

Do you hear the anger at God in those scenarios, the feelings of betrayal? Betrayal is such a painful emotion because it is a betrayal of *trust!* After feeling betrayed, it's very difficult to trust again! As you read the above, you can see why so many Christians are very subtly, and others not so quietly, angry at

God. When I suggest that they might have anger with him, they usually deny it vehemently! And it is not until they are given permission to face and express their anger that some breakthrough begins and they are able to see Jesus weeping. Weeping for them, knocking on the locked door of that area of their wounded heart that contains the hurt and the pain that has been like a poison spilling out from under the door. He is depicted in scripture as *"a man of sorrows and familiar with suffering"*, why? (Isaiah 53:3) As we will explore more, it is clear that we are not living in the world as he created it.

That oozing of pain from beneath our particular locked closet door can affect our lives in countless ways. It can sabotage a desire to be loved by preventing good, healthy relationships, and actually set the person up for further rejection. It can cause a person to procrastinate and not follow through in various situations causing problems in the workplace and at home. It can drive us to succeed in some areas while creating sometimes serious problems in others.

Chuck was very faithful relationally, but when it came to financial provision, he failed his family over and over. Ample income was coming in, but Chuck chose to live only for what satisfied him in the moment – the latest toy or pleasure that drew his attention. He *avoided* facing his financial responsibilities because of some unhealed wounds from the past that had never been faced. It's not unusual to read of many talented CEOs of major companies that have serious relationship problems. How many highly intelligent professors, doctors, or even pastors cannot relate one-on-one with people? Look at the number of marriages so many in the entertainment industry have gone through in spite of their many successes!

One person I am working with I will call Todd. He is a highly successful businessman and admired by many. He's brilliant with his business plans, however Todd continually has major issues relationally, with co-workers, family, friends. He has

CHAPTER 2

blown it off for years, but now it's all catching up with him. As Todd is beginning to have the courage to face his desire for love and connection, he is having to face how the relational pain he experienced as a little boy with his parents is still affecting his relational life today over and over. Todd is also having to acknowledge that no amount of success he's had in business has ever truly satisfied him. He is beginning to recognize that the buried anger erupting in his relationships is coming from the little boy who is still locked up with rage inside him. Todd is also beginning to see the anger the little boy has at God for not saving him from his father. And, he is finally giving himself, and that little boy, permission to be really honest with God. Many of our adult overreactions and problems actually stem from the little child locked within who has never had opportunity to be healed. In many cases, the problems that sabotage our lives, do not begin in the adult, but in the child; however, we do not have to remain trapped within them.

God knows us at the deepest level of our being so he is not surprised or shocked when we finally get gut-level honest with him. If you knew one of your kids was angry at you, wouldn't you rather they be honest with you instead of pretending they're fine and going through the motions? Until they could come clean, you would be relating on the outside, but inside their heart would be closed off. I know that for me as a parent, that would be incredibly sad for I desire heart to heart relationship with my children. God is no different.

That buried pain from the past can prevent us from allowing people to really know us and connect with us on a deep, heart level. Sadly we often deaden even the desire to be loved, accepted, enjoyed, and instead feel more and more rejection because we then draw it unto ourselves. Those feelings of rejection, even if untrue, subtly feed our entitlement of anger. I deadened that desire for acceptance for many years before healing – my motto was, "I don't care", "that doesn't bother me". Both were the lies I told myself, while deep inside I was miserable and desperately desired to be accepted. I just no longer consciously felt anything but indifference because I had tried to kill my desire. Desire doesn't die; it just comes out in ways that are not necessarily life giving, ways that trip us up, like an out of control increasing lust for all sorts of things. We can also carry an atmosphere of anger and rejection that emanates from us without our awareness. That atmosphere pushes people away, while at the same time, we are longing for them to accept us. Then we blame them for not coming close.

Jesus longs to gather us up and pull us in close to his heart. (Isaiah 40:11) He is close to the brokenhearted. (Psalm 34:18) His mission on earth was to heal the brokenhearted. Why? Because we have all been brokenhearted in some way. Broken-heartedness doesn't only come the way Hollywood presents it through a thwarted love story. It happens in everyday life situations when we desire, but then feel snubbed or betrayed. It could be in a job when we feel disregarded or overlooked, or when we feel isolated and alone – like no one cares. The brokenheartedness occurs when we feel unheard and unseen even in our own families, or maybe when life seems to be too much and we are overwhelmed and at the edge of hopelessness and despair. Unfortunately, we don't usually recognize what we are really feeling.

In truth, we often feel what the disciples felt on the Road to Emmaus. The phrase they used often rings true in our own hearts as well, *"I had hoped..."* (Luke 24:13-35). *I had hoped* things would be different, look different, work out differently. *"Hope deferred makes the heart sick, but a longing fulfilled is a tree of life."* (Proverbs 13:12) When our hopes get disappointed, especially in ways concerning our security – areas of need like a job or finances. Or perhaps when special people in our lives reject us, our hearts very often get broken. When we go through a period of experiencing many significant losses during the same timeframe, it becomes a great temptation to lose hope and feel the fingers of despair creep in. However, although it's always possible for us to allow despair to send us on a downward spiral, despair is meant to be a *"door of hope"* for it has a way of breaking all of our lesser hopes. As they go, it leaves us with only one last hope and that is in God himself – *"I am still confident of this; I will see the goodness of The Lord in the land of the living."* (Psalm 27:13).

Healing Takes Place Through Facing Our Reality

For healing to come, we must honestly face our reality. Healing takes place by facing our painful truth, not by running from it. We meet Jesus in our reality, not in our denial. He desires truth in our innermost being as Psalm 51 reminds us. Healing takes place in the light, not by covering over our pain and avoiding it, for he is waiting in the midst of the hurt to meet with us. We have a picture in the gospels of Jesus weeping over Jerusalem, longing to gather them like a hen gathers her chicks, but they were not willing. So often we are not willing to face the hurt that we have locked away either, so he is unable to heal us there. We might have prayed often for our healing, but still not have been willing to cooperate with the process because of a refusal to go back and face our pain. How many times I hear, "Oh, that's in the past!" It might have happened in the past, but it is poisoning our present. Jesus weeps and waits for us to be willing. Just as in obtaining our salvation, he must be invited into our painful emotions. The principle is the same and he is waiting to be allowed into our hurts if deep soul healing is to come.

I have found far too many people, however, unwilling to identify with their pain because then they would no longer be a victim. Sadly, in a twisted way, victimhood can become a false identity or hiding place. When, for a long time, we have lived as a victim of some hurtful act done to us as a child, it can become something we are familiar with, almost comfortable with, and it can be difficult to release it. We unfortunately *know how to be a victim*, but we don't yet know how to live without that false identity. I lived as a victim of my pain for far too many years and it sabotaged my life! *"But you, O God, do see trouble and grief; you consider it to take it in hand. The victim commits himself to you, you are the helper of the fatherless."* (Psalm 10:14)

The World in Which We Were Originally Created to Live

This is not the world God originally created. He created the Garden, a place of love, tenderness, harmony and peace, not fear. A place of belonging, of feeling valued, wanted, and enjoyed. God created man with a dependent spirit for man to need him, to walk with him, and to have purpose. He put man in the garden to lovingly tend it in his own unique way with the gifts and talents he placed within him. The breath of God in the clay Adam was formed from gave him life. His being was not independent of God but instead dependent on him for life that would be full of rich purpose. As a result, Adam and Eve were able to co-labor with God in the Garden without stress or toil in great freedom and joy. They were naked (exposed) but without any shame or fear of failure. (Genesis 2)

What happened to that life? The Fall. The choice of man, tempted by the enemy, to do things their own way instead of God's. The subtle suggestion by the enemy was that God was holding out on them, that he really didn't have their best interest in mind, so they'd best take matters into their own hands and do it their own way. The temptation was that they could be *like* God Himself by being their *own* god and knowing good and evil. It's interesting to note that until they listened to the snake and ate from the wrong tree, there was no evil that they had to contend with. Even in their

CHAPTER 2

nakedness, they felt no shame because they were covered with God's light and glory.

However all that changed with their agreement of the enemy's lure to eat from the wrong tree, and so Adam and Eve began the difficult journey of the life we all struggle with today. Things like pride, shame, blame, selfishness, fear, toil, hurt, pain, fearing exposure by covering over and avoiding – basically hiding their true selves. We find the beginnings of fear, anger, jealousy, and even murder entering the scene. And this is just at the beginning of the story in chapters 3 and 4 of Genesis. The loss of true life starts right in the beginning of man's history as a result of their choice to no longer be dependent on God for life, but instead chose life for themselves, in their own way. It was their Independence Day, but with horrible results for the entire world right to this day. Sadly God gets blamed over and over for the horrific consequences of man's choice to be his own god.

Even their work was meant to be full of life and peaceful garden tending, but instead it became demanding, toiling, striving, stressing and never really enough to fully satisfy. Sometimes we think it does, especially when the compensation is good, but we are not aware of what the perfect was meant to be. No wonder we carry a deep dissatisfaction within. We settle for it as normal because we have been so far removed from God's original high intentions and design. As our Creator, no wonder Jesus is spoken of as a "man of sorrows", for he knows who we were originally created to be.

Right in the beginning of the story in Gen. 6:5,6, God gives us a picture of his broken heart as he looked at the evil that grew out of man's decision to be his own god and do things in his own way. *"The Lord saw how great man's wickedness on the earth had become, and that every inclination of the thoughts of his heart was only evil all the time. The Lord was grieved that he had made man on the earth, and his heart was filled with pain."* Have you ever thought of God's heart being broken and filled with pain? That's why he sent Jesus to give his life for us so we could begin to walk in the redemption of the life we were eternally meant to live. Once we are willing to truly journey with him in his way, and allow him access to heal our previously broken hearts, we can begin to cooperate in living little by little from the new heart Jesus paid for. That good heart is meant to go on for all eternity. (Ezekiel 36:26-27)

By living in this broken world as a man who experienced every temptation we do and every painful emotion we struggle with ourselves, Jesus knows our pain firsthand. He too was rejected, despised, abused, mocked, ridiculed, left all alone at the worst time of his life, denied by one of his closest friends, and betrayed by another. Jesus longed for his friends to understand his anguish just as we do. Feeling overwhelmed to the point of sweating blood, he struggled with powerlessness the same as we. He wrestled with his Father, begging him to take the cup he was facing from him. Why did Jesus have to suffer all of those emotions? Because we do – how else could he be a faithful high priest who understands our struggle, making the way for our restoration? He went all the way through to the end to make a way for us – for heaven, thankfully yes, but also for us to be restored to his original intent for our lives.

He longs to fulfill his mission *in* us to *"bind up the brokenhearted, to proclaim freedom for the captives and release from darkness for the prisoners"* since we have all become captives to a very broken world. (Isaiah 61:1) *"The Lord is close to the brokenhearted and saves those who are crushed in spirit"* (Psalm 34:18). Those are not just nice words on a page, but as we finally become willing to enter our pain with him, they truly become our reality and restored life!

CHAPTER 2

The Two Trees in the Garden of Eden

If eating from the wrong tree, the Tree of the Knowledge of Good and Evil in the Garden was so devastating for all of us, maybe we should take a look at the differences between the two trees God put in the Garden to test them. The two trees produce two very different paradigms of living. From the first tree, the Tree of the Knowledge of Good and Evil, comes the world system, a system of power and control that puts man at the center. Unfortunately far too much of the church is based on this system even though the appearance is given of God being first and foremost. Notice there is both a good and an evil side. When we eat from that tree we might insist that it's only from the good side we are dining. We might *pride* ourselves in declaring we would never eat from the evil side, but even the *good* of that tree is illusion; it's religion and not true life. Jesus made the statement that only God is good. All our own goodness is as filthy rags, the Scripture reminds us, so let's look at the different fruit produced by each tree.

The Tree of the Knowledge of Good and Evil

From the Tree of the Knowledge of Good and Evil comes illusion, pretense, the need to wear a mask and strive to be acceptable. It requires perfectionism and performance in order to prove ourselves worthy and acceptable. It feeds and covers our shame with *"fig leaves"* and produces our pride. It is toiling, but not restful garden tending. It causes fear, anxiety, control, ungodly competition, anger, demandingness, the need to prove oneself, and to protect ourselves at any expense from the possibility of any failure that might be lurking. It begins with self and not with God, although God might be added on. Within the church he is usually the first add on, but yet our life still begins with us, and not with him. I believe a majority of born again believers, who will go to heaven when they die, are currently still eating from the wrong tree without realizing it. That is the tree of religion.

With that tree we try to prove ourselves valuable through what we *do* instead of who we *are*. Whether we use our education, career, success, motherhood, family, ministry, athletics, popularity, material possessions, status, power, or any other thing to get our worth, we are still eating from the wrong tree. Living from this tree traps us in an identity of shame, causing a fear of experiencing any future shame and being discovered as a failure. We may secretly feel we are never enough. It feeds the usually buried lie that we don't measure up and fear being found out as not having what it takes. This is the essence of the lie that is at the root of our buried shame. Although each person usually has their own words to describe that false belief, in their thoughts, they will usually fluctuate between thinking of themselves as less than others or more than other people.

For the latter, the shame lie drives them to pride and they feel better than everyone else, often secretly looking down on others. I have found that the ones who view themselves as more than others can have a harder time seeing their lie of shame and it sometimes takes a huge crisis of exposure to break through that lie, as was the case of someone I recently met with. He prided himself in what he did, got his identity from it, and then out of the blue he was fired! It was such a devastating blow that his whole identity crumbled in a moment. (I will share more on both legitimate and illegitimate shame in chapter four.)

A close friend of mine gave me permission to share his story with you in the hopes you would understand the gravity of circumstances that can come from not quickly facing any shame lies you might have buried inside. My friend, who is extremely intelligent, creative, capable, and a Christian with a good heart, built his survival system on the pride side of feeling better than others. No matter how much we talked about shame, he never seemed to recognize that his pride and arrogance was being driven by a false shame belief about himself that took hold early on through some very painful circumstances. Unfortunately, it took the horrifically shameful, major crisis of prison to bring my friend to his knees before he was finally able to identify the lie that had driven his entire life. As a result of the denial and his not being willing to go to the root of his problems earlier, the whole family was tremendously hurt through the resulting circumstances in ways too numerous to count.

However, I am also extremely overjoyed to see how God is daily taking what the enemy meant for evil in his life, and using it for good, even though the resulting consequences continue to be painful for them all. I share this story to encourage you to do whatever it takes and invite the Spirit to help you identify any shame beliefs you might be carrying. Without even realizing it, those false beliefs might be affecting your daily life, your future life, and the lives of those you care about as well. Don't wait until the crisis comes!

Another example is someone I will call Jen who threw her whole life into motherhood to the point of controlling her children's every move. She was going to have them turn out right and prove to whomever she was a good mother. Sadly, it was never about loving her children well, but instead about *proving herself* a great mother. Unfortunately, as her children reached adulthood, they were incapable of living their own lives in a healthy manner. Each reacted differently, but they were all crippled and unable to become the emotionally healthy adults they were meant to be.

The Tree of Life

When, instead, we begin the journey to consciously feed on the Tree of Life, we begin a mission with Jesus of life-giving co-labor with his purposes. It first gives life to us, then overflows from out of our inner being, that which is in harmony with Jesus' life, to others. However, the life that comes out through us is not just generic life, it is uniquely ours! It comes from the person Jesus knew before we were ever born, the person he created uniquely and wonderfully before the robbery of a broken world ever happened to us. (Psalm 139) We begin to discover the person Jesus knew even before our parents did, the one who got lost under our performance, our trying to be acceptable. And as we cooperate with the life the Spirit of Jesus breathes into us, we are molded within our own unique personality, with our own particular gifts, our history, including even the brokenness that we are allowing him to redeem. As a result, once again we become *living beings,* bringing forth his life to a hurting world through our own uniqueness in the way prepared for us to walk in. *"For we are God's workmanship, created in Christ Jesus to do good works, which God prepared in advance for us to do."* (Ephesians 2:10)

The Tree of Life is Jesus. He is the way, the truth, and the Life and the only way to life that's really life! He is the truth about life no matter what the world may tell us. It's from him we draw our life with joy from the well of salvation. (Isaiah 12:3) It's like putting an empty bucket into a well and drawing up the water. That well of living water is within us. It's Jesus living his life from inside us, through us, yet with our own submission of will, beauty, and uniqueness. He is not far off, he is closer than our breath – in fact he is the breath of our life when we join with him. One of the things Jesus did after his resurrection was to breathe on his disciples, giving them back the breath of true life that was lost through the Fall.

When we live in him, drawing from his life within us, we are never alone because we are joined to another who is brimming with life in the depth of our being. The process for each of us though, is learning to abide with him there, learning to flow from his life within us instead of instinctively from our own ways and demanding hearts. It is a process of awareness first, then a conscious drawing of his life from within us. I used to always feel alone, even in a crowd, but as I have been learning to draw my life from his within me, I don't feel alone anymore because I am not.

When we have lived a life connected to the way that seemed right to us, we far too often never realized that way was not life producing, but instead brought a form of death to us even while we lived! Our own way is always the more comfortable way, the broad way instead of the narrow one that few Christians ever truly discover. However he is calling to each of us to join him on his journey for us instead of our own. Jesus' way for us takes our being willing to die to that old familiar way we lived, even as Christians, in order to fully live out our lives with him by collaborating with his purposes. Drawing life from this tree eventually causes us to willingly give up ourselves and our own agendas by tuning into what he is doing and joining him in it. That's the life Jesus lived – he only did what he saw his Father doing. From this tree, it's not about us anymore, but about working with him to fulfill his purposes through us in the way we were uniquely designed.

Then we begin to become authentic life-givers, walking in integrity and peace of heart and mind. We begin to discover our true identity and worth, no longer living from fear of shame, but from the life of Jesus within us. Our cooperation with his life in us produces peace, joy, rest, as well as released creativity that comes from *the* Creator himself who is living inside us. We begin to learn how to abide, remaining in him, drawing from his life within instead of our own. *"With joy you will draw water from the well of salvation."* (Isaiah 12:3) Our character begins to change as a result and the fruit of his Spirit begins to grow. He has created us for adventure so life begins to be exciting instead of dull, especially as we join him on the journey he has prepared for us – the one that fits us in with how we were uniquely designed. We begin to be led from the center of our being where Jesus is. Directed from a center of grace and peace, instead of "should's" and "ought to's", so there becomes a life-giving flow instead of false guilt and stress.

Instead of *human doings*, we begin to become authentic *human beings*. Our *being* coming out of the great *I AM* himself. Years ago when I was struggling with all this, he made the statement to me, *"Because I AM, you are"*. Wow! That is where our true substance, security, stability, and identity comes from – the powerful, Almighty, I Am of God who is pleased to dwell within us. He is the God who is always there, continually alive, constantly present and no matter what our struggle or circumstance may look like, HE IS! He is *not, I will be or I was*, but the ever present *I AM!* Of course, we must remember that learning to abide and draw from his life within us is a journey with him, a process that continually produces life in us as long as we remain connected. At any point we are free to jump ship and return to living from that wrong tree. This new journey comes through learning to draw life from the presence of God within and then beginning to recognize when we have gone back again to living from the wrong center. It requires staying in touch with our own hearts!

Jesus' end-time prayer in John 17 was that we would be *united* with him, that we would be *one* with him. That's not just meant to be a nice religious picture, but a *secret of true life* – the life that's really life, peace, joy, and fulfillment of purpose – the purpose for which we were created comes from remaining united! Colossians 1:27 gives us the key, *"Christ in us the hope of glory"*. Our lives begin to take on powerful purpose when we begin to live from our Divine center where Christ is. John 15 gives us a beautiful picture of this in Jesus' illustration of the vine and the branches, so much so, that Jesus reminds us that *without him we can do nothing*. Oh we do lots of things, busy stuff, but anything we do of eternal value or true significance must come out of the life of God within us. Those are the things that will never be

CHAPTER 2

burned up and will remain eternally. (1 Corinthians 3:11-14) I don't know about you, but my heart cry is that I will co-labor with him in bearing fruit that will last for all eternity!

CHAPTER 3
Finding God's Peace in the Struggles of Our Lives

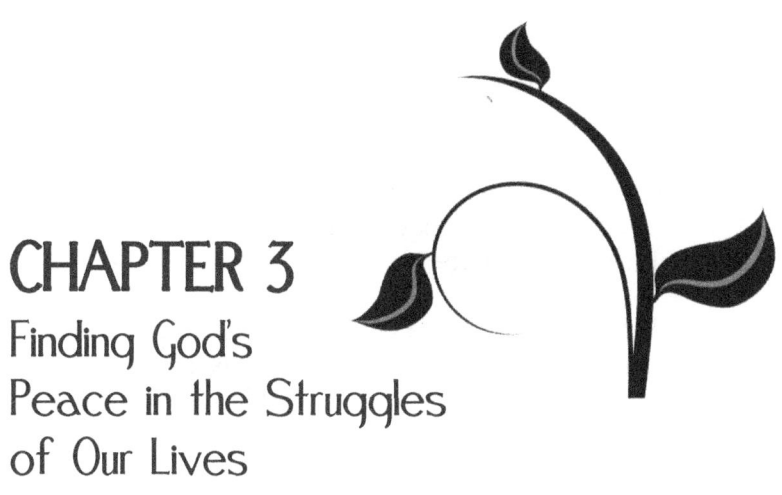

Have you ever noticed God doesn't necessarily do things the way we would? Just like the story of Jesus in Mark 4:35-41 when Jesus led his disciples into a *storm* – why would he do that? We sometimes have a picture that there should be no storm if Jesus is on board our little boat. However that was not the case when Jesus gave the invitation to his disciples, those he loved, to go into the boat over to the other side of the lake with him. He then proceeded to fall asleep on a cushion! A storm began to brew on the water that was so full of fury, raging all around them and creating such terror in his disciples' hearts that they were horrified of drowning. Their cry was one we can relate to for sure, *"Teacher, don't you care if we drown?"*

Jesus led my husband and I into a storm when we bought our condo. It was apparent the time had come for us to move because our house had become far too much for us to handle and the Spirit had confirmed that clearly to both of our hearts. We had a good practice of never making a major move until we were both in one accord with what we felt the Lord was saying, so we finally bought a For Sale sign. After having it in the garage for a while, one evening around eight o'clock, my husband Bruce, felt God saying it was time to put

CHAPTER 3

the sign in the front yard. By seven-thirty the following morning, a neighbor jogged by, saw the sign, went home and called us with a request to buy the house! This all unbelievably took place in less than twelve nighttime hours. We discovered the condo we were interested in was still available, and upon entering it, we had tremendous peace and a knowing that it was the one, so we bought it. It probably wasn't even three weeks after moving in, when to our dismay, we discovered there was a lawsuit pending with the entire association that would double our maintenance payment each month!

We deeply struggled when that fact was revealed, my husband getting mostly angry, but I instead had fear and the terrifying question – had we not heard God? Did we miss it completely? If we had, then what about all the other times we thought we had heard God – did we really? Much doubt and confusion entered, and on top of that, what about the increased maintenance fee; we hadn't budgeted for that! Where was God? Asleep on a cushion? As I was willing to enter the struggle and wrestle out my fears with God, I heard him tell me that it was *his storm*. OK, so if it was his storm, then he wasn't surprised by the lawsuit and somehow he would provide the extra money needed each month, which he did. A strange peace replaced the struggle and that lesson changed my paradigm of God's ways in a tremendously meaningful way. God has used a storm in the lives of so many I have worked with in order to change their way of interpreting life and the way they believed God was obligated to act on their behalf. Isaiah 55:9 reminds us that, *"As the heavens are higher than the earth so are my ways higher than your ways and my thoughts than your thoughts."*

Even though we know that verse is true, when God doesn't act in the way we had thought he would, there usually is an emotional reaction, and yet the tendency with too many Christians is to just bury their angst. *"After all God is God, right? – What's the point in wrestling with it? He always wins!"*

The point is that our emotions are the voice of our hearts and our hearts matter to God. When we ignore what our hearts are feeling, we are simply burying our emotions. Then we can begin to feel strangely distant from God, get angry at him, or get into a mode of pretense that everything is fine when it's not because now our hearts are shut down. We go through the motions, but our hearts are actually far from him. We often get offended with God. In reality though, God often offends our minds and our own understanding in order to get to the beliefs really buried in our hearts! When we are willing to wrestle through our struggle with God, he is able to listen to our voice, and is always understanding of our fear. Then as we begin to feel seen and heard again, he feels safer, and it becomes easier to surrender to his ways. As a result, he is able to lift us up to a higher level of trust in him.

The Different Seasons of Our Lives

"There is a time for everything, and a season for every activity under heaven;..." (Ecclesiastes 3:1)

When life the way we have built it begins to fall apart, our first natural response is usually anger or anxiety. *"Where is God? Why isn't he protecting me?"* Those might be the feelings we have, if not the exact words we would use. The Christian life has various seasons just like we find in nature. Some are seasons of blessing and enjoyment where we seemingly can do no wrong. It's just like the warm *"south wind"* referred to in Song of Solomon, but occasionally we will experience a *"north wind"* of adversity, a season that feels like a very cold, harsh northern winter where the winds never seem to stop and there is one bone-chilling blizzard after another. In that season, we often experience problem after problem. Just as we begin to recover from one, another happens, and occasionally they happen in various areas all at once! We begin to feel like we have been beaten up!

CHAPTER 3

It can sometimes feel like we are a tree being chopped down with blow after blow. There might be a variety of crisis situations happening one after another without reprieve – different things for different people. The struggles we might be facing could be almost anything – like the breakdown of a necessary vehicle, a flood in the home through faulty plumbing, one financial crisis after another, health issues that seem unsolvable, various relationship problems – some very serious, ongoing situations with children or teens, issues on the job or even job loss. The list goes on and on. Sometimes this scriptural picture from Amos 5:19 is descriptive of what it feels like in that season, *"It will be as though a man fled from a lion only to meet a bear, as though he entered his house and rested his hand on the wall only to have a snake bite him"*.

The things that happen are very personal for each of us, but the feelings we experience are often the same. Feelings of fear of the losses involved, emotions of abandonment and feeling forsaken even when we know in our heads it isn't true. At that time the enemy usually whispers in our hearts that God has forsaken us and that our troubles will never end, but it's crucial we recognize those condemning words as the lie they are. It is a painfully purposeful season, but only a season. In Hosea 2:15, God reveals that the *"Valley of Achor"* (trouble) is meant to become *"a door of hope"*. Rev. S. Chadwick in the little old devotional book, Streams in the Desert, states that *"Desperation is better than despair"* because, *"the wit's end of desperation was the beginning of God's power"* and *"are the stepping stones in the path of light"*.

In my walk through that discouragingly painful season of adversity that the north wind brought, the Spirit encouraged me with Scripture from Isaiah 28 where he paints a picture of hope. The verses describe a farmer plowing the ground in order to plant a crop, but reminds us that the farmer doesn't plow forever, only enough to sow his seed. Then in verse 28, he gives us the end result of the whole process, *"Grain must *be ground to make bread so one does not go on threshing it forever".* God desires to make bread out of our lives, our particular flavor of bread, but that bread must first be broken *in us* before it can truly feed anyone else. That is a huge part of the difficult winter season we go through – he takes us, breaks the natural way in us, so that what comes forth after the grinding feeds both ourselves and others! Someone I know would always laughingly say when referring to that season, "God's got me in the grinder!"

What else are those seasons about and where is God when we need him so badly? Isaiah 30:20 gives us a picture of what God desires to have come out of the adversity and affliction. Paraphrased, it tells us that our teachers will not be hidden anymore and we will develop such an intimacy with him that we will more clearly hear his voice directing us. That season is meant to create a desperate dependency upon him in us on levels we didn't even know were possible.

Much good in us happens through those confusing seasons, that at the time, feel so empty and dark. The wilderness season purifies our hearts. Without realizing it, too many times we have a divided heart. Part of me does and part of me doesn't. Psalm 86:11 says, *"Teach me your way, O Lord and I will walk in your truth; give me an undivided heart that I may fear your name".* This dark season of what can sometimes even feel like despair brings the mixture of our hearts to the surface because our survival systems are no longer working and that is slowly causing us to become more and more unglued. It feels terrible to experience the undoing of our old ways, but necessary if we are to learn to trust God and truly become who we were originally created to be. The end result is an ability to experience the joy of living a life that is really life!

In the wilderness season God is often tearing down things in us we didn't even realize were there, or if we did, saw nothing wrong with them. It could be something like a false picture of God and his ways, as I had before my condo experience. It might be a demand that God come through for us in a particular way – our own way, the way we desperately thought things needed to work out if we were to feel ok and survive. Or perhaps he might be tearing down the particular survival systems we have erected. We look to them for life – things like our performance, our perfectionism, the security of a job, or the need to make significant relationships work in order to feel secure and have our lives continue the way we need them to be.

Before the shaking of our systems, we are usually totally unaware those things are not the true security we are looking to experience. That's why nothing has been ever enough to fill the insatiable need inside, or that there is even anything wrong with the way we are believing. Many people have already shut their deep desires down and are no longer even aware of their hungry heart – they have simply settled. Our families might have handled life that way for generations, so it is our normal or standard and it feels right. However, erecting our own particular survival system is often a way of controlling or at least trying to control our own lives in order to feel safe and secure. In that case, we become our *own* god instead of entrusting our lives and futures into God's hands and sadly, those systems become our idols. *"Just as I watched over them to uproot and tear down, and to overthrow, destroy and bring disaster, so I will watch over them to build and to plant, declares The Lord."* (Jeremiah 31:28) What is he tearing down, destroying? Simply our own systems, our own way of trying to make life the way we feel it must if we are to feel secure and satisfied. That is the wrong foundation and it must come down if we are to find our true selves.

However, strangely enough, while we are overwhelmingly experiencing those undoing feelings, we can at the same time, begin to recognize a faint peace coming from somewhere very deep in our hearts that makes no sense at all. Strangely, out of our struggle, comes a birthing of the *"peace of God which transcends all understanding"* referred to in Philippians 4:7. Notice it says the peace *of* God – that is the peace coming from Christ himself who is living his life on the inside of us. He is still in control even as our own control is destructing all around us, causing us to feel like our world, as we've arranged it, is crumbling. And in fact our created world is crumbling, but through it, we begin to see that he is truly the Rock under our feet. *"He is before all things, and in him all things hold together."* (Colossians 1:17)

It has been my experience and the experience of many others that, in the midst of that seemingly destructive season, when we need God most to enter and put a stop to things, he seems to be strangely absent. I experienced a year like that a number of years ago. At the time, what seemed like one of the worst years of my life, as I now look back, I realize it was one of the most life changing years. I never want to go through it again, but my whole view of life has had a tremendous readjustment as a result of that horrible year. I have walked with countless others through the years with the same experience. In fact I hear a similar story over and over from those who have walked or are currently walking through their own confusing, mostly dark, wilderness season. In that painful season God redoes the foundations our lives have been built upon, as well as very often adjusts even our understanding of things we previously thought we understood. Things like God, love, marriage, family, friendships, faith, church, work, and generally just life itself. After going through that difficult period myself, I found I had to ask God to redefine all those things to me from his perspective.

In the wilderness season when all seems to have dried up, we often feel abandoned and alone, sometimes even forsaken by God and those we care about most – it's like we are on the backside of the desert. The picture is very similar to the journey the Israelites went through in the wilderness those

CHAPTER 3

forty years, but thankfully ours is not meant to last for anywhere near that long. Why do we have to go through that? Deuteronomy 8:2-3 gives as a clue as to what it some of it is about. *"Remember how The Lord your God led you all the way in the desert these forty years to humble you and to test you in order to know what was in your heart, whether you would keep his commands. He humbled you, causing you to hunger and then feeding you with manna, which neither you nor your fathers had known, to teach you man does not live on bread alone but on every word that comes from the mouth of The Lord."*

It is in that place where nothing seems to work the way we need it to, a desperate dependency upon God is developed. Unfortunately that kind of dependency often only comes after we have allowed ourselves to get very real with God, even angry and maybe allowing ourselves a bit of a tantrum! I have had many tantrums over the years as I struggled to learn that God's ways are really far superior to mine even though I couldn't always see it at the time.

Let me share another powerful quote with you from the devotional, <u>Streams in the Desert</u>, *"Beloved, do not try to get out of a dark place, except in God's time and way. The time of trouble is meant to teach you lessons that you sorely need. Premature deliverance may frustrate God's work of grace in your life. Just commit the whole situation to him..."*

One pastor I was meeting with was trapped in a desert season with a lot of buried anger. As much as he loved God, he also hated him for the abuse he had suffered as a child and in order to get unstuck from that ambivalence, he had to allow his rage to surface in a way that didn't harm anyone else. As a result, he was at last able to expose the words he had been harboring in his heart so they could finally be released. As he was eventually able to wrestle with the hurts and false beliefs that were trapped beneath his anger, he uncovered a passion for God and his kingdom of which he was previously unaware. This young man has an amazing gift that, I believe, can now be released more and more to touch a lost world and awaken a sleeping church.

If you were to renovate your house, there would have to be a tearing out of the old before the new could be built – even walls might have to come down. I enjoy watching those home shows where they come in and mercilessly tear down a house to its studs. The mess is overwhelming and the dumpster full of useless debris, but for the new to be built, the old must go. They don't rebuild on top of the rotten wood, it must all be removed. And even worse, as they proceed, more and more rotten wood is sometimes uncovered that often prolongs the rebuilding process. How often they think they have finally torn out the last of the rottenness only to find a whole other section still to be removed. As I was praying for a couple whose marriage was in trouble recently, God showed me their marriage had originally been built on anger and fear so their foundation was faulty. It had to come down! That didn't mean the marriage was over, only that the tearing down had to happen so the foundation could be rebuilt.

So with us, God must tear out the old – those ways of our own survival, the controlling structures we have built to make life work out our own way, the way that seemed right at the time, but actually brought death instead of life. Places in us we didn't even realize were just "rotten wood" have to come down so there is a good foundation for the new, the real to be erected on. You can't put truth on top of a lie and expect it to remain. The lies, the false beliefs, have to be exposed as the "rotten wood" they are, so the new can stand. *"There is a way that seems right to a man, but in the end it leads to death."* (Proverbs 16:25)

One couple I met with individually watched as bit by bit both of their personal worlds as well as their marriage, seemed to be crumbling, and unfortunately almost every major area of

CHAPTER 3

their lives felt like it was being affected. The good life, the way they had designed it, just wasn't happening. Their marriage didn't seem to be working and they couldn't agree on much of anything anymore. It felt as if God was angry and had forgotten them, but he wasn't, he didn't. He was desiring to rebuild their lives on a new foundation of peace and love instead of their trying to make life work their own way and according to their blueprint. It felt as if they personally, as well as their marriage, would be destroyed as it was all happening, but they weren't – instead they came out the other side as changed people. In place of the destruction they feared, as they finally gave up the struggle against God and were at last able to surrender themselves individually to God and his ways, things began to turn.

At long last, in desperation they began to embrace the "crazy" thing the Spirit seemed to be doing in their lives; even though it didn't seem right and they no longer claimed to understand his ways. I have heard countless people come out of this season with more questions than answers, saying, "I no longer know what I thought I knew!" But as they became more willing to release it all to God, almost immediately there was a turning of circumstances. Although it was almost imperceptible at first, and though it never looked like they originally thought it would, it was truly for good. As a result, they found themselves on a deeper level of relationship both with each other and with God, as well as discovering a level of peace in the bigger picture they never knew existed. As they began to flow with God in his ways instead of their own, their difficult circumstances somehow began working out as well.

"And we know that in all things God works for the good of those who love him, who have been called according to his purpose." (Romans 8:28)

In the process of restoring relationship, each had to be willing to enter a deep heart struggle to give up their anger at each other and also with God for seemingly not answering their prayers. They began to see that their false pictures and demands didn't originate in the marriage, but went back to childhood hurts and past relational disappointments – they just played out in the marriage. As they were willing to allow God to heal those places in their own hearts where the past hurts caused the demands to begin, God began to restore the marriage and rebuild their family. This continues to be a process for them that takes vulnerability and courage instead of blame. For true change to come, they had to be willing to face themselves along with their disappointed desires, forgive each other, and be willing to take the log out of their own eye first.

Another couple had to face the tremendous uncertainty and fear they felt because of some bad life-altering decisions their children had made out of their own rebellion. Through trying to fix their children's problems, their house was now under foreclosure. Their present lack of security also threatened their health because of the stress, and the list went on and on. To come to the peace that passes understanding, they had to meet God as their only true security in each area in a whole new way. It was a way that went to the depth of their being and was not just a Sunday religion. They began to recognize that Jesus is their only true hope for life and that truly, "He will be the sure foundation for their times...", in a whole new way (Isaiah 33:6). I am excited that every time I see them, I see a new depth of real life and joy emanating from them even though, at times, they still struggle with each other.

We Live with Mixture

There is real mixture in true life because of the broken world we live in and it's necessary for us to embrace that. We can silently demand black or white, all or nothing, but that will never fully be realized until we see Jesus face to face. In the meantime we live with both gifts and losses at the same time. The more we are willing to honestly face and mourn our losses, the more we are able to recognize tiny gifts we would have otherwise missed. The exciting acknowledgement of those sometimes small gifts develops a thankful heart within us for they are now able to bring us joy, sometimes right in the midst of our sorrow.

The false beliefs that have driven us have often come out of our buried fears and lack of trust in God and his good heart in taking care of us. Sometimes we just are driven from our silent demands that life work out our own way, the way we think we need it to. That belief system comes from the wrong tree, the Tree of the Knowledge of Good and Evil. It's how our own understanding and knowledge tells us life should be working for us. When it does all work, we feel safe and secure, but when God thwarts us in it, we feel like our lives are falling apart. Actually, what is crumbling is not us, but our control, our system of making life work out our own way. In that case our survival system has been our security, not God, so he begins to shake us and as he does, the wrongly-built foundations of our lives begin to quake! We are reminded in Proverbs 3:5 that we are to trust in him, and not lean on our own knowledge and understanding. Then when we do trust, even though it feels frightening at times, our paths are directed by a loving Father. We have given up our independent spirit and exchanged it for a desperate dependency upon God.

We don't feel particularly loved while our world appears to be crumbling. It feels much more like God is against us, but he is not. He's actually loving us well in not allowing us to continue to build our lives on that false foundation, and that which we have tried to hold together will probably eventually crumble anyway. Sadly, even if we do manage to survive with our systems intact, we will never taste the true security and real peace that remains even in the midst of the storms of life, or the rest in him he desires we daily experience no matter what our circumstances happen to be.

By finally letting go, we delightfully discover that his yoke is truly easy and his burden light as we learn little by little to remain in the yoke with him, co-laboring in the way he prepared for us. (Matthew 11:28-30) If God does not shake our own created world, we will sadly continue to sabotage the life that truly satisfies and never fully taste the experiences and purposes we were created to enjoy with him. Instead we will hug the shore or make impulsive mistakes, but either way, limp through life with fear, anger, control, and anxiety. God's joyful desire for us is that we experience peace at the deepest level of our inner being and move together with him in harmony.

"The words once more indicate the removing of what can be shaken--that is, the created things – so that what cannot be shaken may remain." (Hebrews 12:27) Notice that it is our *"created things"* that get shaken. In other words, the systems of life that we have created in order to survive. When they come down, God can rebuild our lives on his foundation of love and true security.

Why do we resist a life so wonderful? We can look at several reasons. One, it is frightening for us to feel out of control and powerless especially if we have experienced being out of control and alone in our powerlessness as a child. The only way we can surrender a fear that overpowering is to be able to trust God on a deep heart level and believe he has a good, caring, and involved heart toward us. Two, painful circumstances we have lived through caused by significant people failing us, betraying us, rejecting us through the years have taught our hearts that its foolish to trust and just let go – we'd better hold our own world together or it will collapse! Three, we inherited the desire for control from our original parents, Adam and Eve. Demanding the knowledge of what is going to happen next can be control. Too often we silently

CHAPTER 3

demand to know the end from the beginning. We want to have full understanding of the journey in between which leaves us feeling more in control and not just having to helplessly trust in God. Once again we are trying to live our lives from the wrong tree of independence instead of from dependence upon Jesus, the Tree of Life.

Just the other day I had someone struggling with that control and a demand to know and understand why God was allowing all that he was. After all, it was unfair! We couldn't seem to get past that point until I, without thinking, just blurted out, "You're eating from the wrong tree!" That grabbed him and seemed to bring some disruption to his demand to understand. The truth is, many times we will not understand God's ways for they are higher than ours. We can't bring him down to our way of seeing, we must be willing to go up to his and a gradual, sometimes painfully slow, relearning of his ways.

I have watched countless people, including myself at times, hold on to the way we think is right until our knuckles are white! To let go would feel like the destruction of everything we hold near and dear. I have learned the hard way that the more I've tried to make things work the way I thought they needed to, the more God in his great love for me simply thwarted my plans. The more I banged on the door, the silence on the other side was deafening, and God seemed like he was nowhere to be found. However, as I was finally willing to struggle through from a deep place in my heart in surrender to God and to his ways, a peace began to flood my soul. Then in his timing things began to reorder.

Early on my journey of surrender instead of control, the Spirit of God gave me a vision. I saw myself as a very little girl (the age I was when my ability to trust was first robbed from me) and I was on an extremely winding path with Jesus. There was Florida jungle on either side of the path and he had just one request of me. Jesus simply and kindly, said,

"Hold my hand, I am the way". Because I was at a very young age on this journey, I did as little children often do, I dropped his hand. Time and time again I found myself lost in the jungle with panic in my heart, screaming out, *"Jesus, I'm lost!"* Jesus' response to me was always the same – very lovingly he simply left the path, picked me up out of the jungle, brushed me off, smiled and said, *"Hold my hand"*. There was never a rebuke for my actions, he simply invited me to stay connected to him by holding his hand so I wouldn't get lost...

But then I would look ahead, see the bend on the path, feel the terror in the pit of my stomach regarding what might unexpectedly be lurking around the next curve... However once again his loving response simply was, *"I know what's there, you just have to hold my hand to remain safe. Remember that I am the way"*. I was stuck in this vision for at least three months. As we went over and over it through various circumstances and fears, I finally became able to trust him more and more without panic when I looked at my future and the many uncertainties that were going on in my life at that time. Up to that time, I had always lived my life just waiting for the next shoe to drop! However in that new season of learning to trust, even though my circumstances seemed hopeless, through his gentleness I began to learn that he indeed was my way through. And then from there I had to learn that he was also my truth, and finally that Christ in me was my life! (Colossians 1:27)

Through that season I learned to write my letters to God each day. My fears of letting go were overwhelming! As I poured out my honest struggle to him, he began to speak back to me with words of encouragement, strength, peace, and even loving correction that instead of either shaming or devastating me, brought life and hope. A new intimacy and re-fathering, re-mothering began to happen, one in which I felt loved and secure. *"Though my father and mother forsake me, The Lord will receive me."* (Psalm 27:10) I've encouraged many to share their struggling hearts with him in this way and at first, I often hear things like, "I'm not a writer like you – I don't even like to write". That's ok because I didn't at first either, but it was a lifeline for my sinking ship and through it I developed an incredible love of writing to him. In fact, it's usually the part of my time with him that brings the most connection, first with my own heart, then with his. I encourage you to get honest with your heart as well, including Jesus in that struggle you are in the midst of. He is waiting for you there.

I am including some very brief excerpts below from my letters to God that, especially in the early days, sometimes were as many as twelve to fourteen pages as I poured my heart out to him in my struggles. I share so you can know you're not alone in your angst and struggle. One person I met with, who probably resisted my suggestion to write letters to God the most with various excuses, one day began and to this day often gets up at four or five in the morning to write her pages to him. It has become a lifeline for her heart as well.

My Struggle:
My Father, I am feeling so alone and forgotten, lonely, forsaken even by those around me. Where are you? – it feels like you have forgotten me too. I am feeling overwhelmed and yet even you seem afar off and silent. My feelings are like those in Psalm 31:12 "I am forgotten by them as though I were dead; I have become like broken pottery." 14,15... "But I trust in you, O Lord; I say, 'You are my God'. My times are in your hands..."

God's Response to Me:

"My child, your journey of aloneness must be walked with me. I am your higher way of life and I will walk you through to the other side. As I walked with Jesus in his aloneness so I will walk with you. Aloneness is good for the soul and necessary for healing from your wound of abandonment. But it is also hard and painful because it is not a shared experience and feels too close to the original abandonment you experienced. This valley must be walked through in isolation, feeling alone, but never alone, just as Jesus was not alone in his isolation experience, for I was with him. (John 16:32) As I was with Jesus so I am with you in your alone place. It is only on your journey through the aloneness that you discover the reality of the words that now bring you comfort, but are not yet truth in the depths of your being. True peace, rest, and security come only through my meeting with you there in that alone and empty place. Enter that place with me; do not run from it!"

My Struggle:

Father, so many hard things are happening that I am feeling totally overwhelmed. It seems like the problems will never end. Where are you, do you see? I need you so desperately, please enter this world of adversity I feel trapped in. Thanks. "Although The Lord gives you the bread of adversity and the water of affliction, your teachers will be hidden no more, with your own eyes you will see them. Whether you turn to the right or to the left, your ears will hear a voice behind you saying, 'This is the way, walk in it.'" (Isaiah 30:20-21)

God's Response to Me:

"My child, true deep internal breakthrough often comes through adversity. Your genuine human neediness that comes *from past and present unmet emotional and spiritual hunger has to surface from where it has been buried in your heart. Then it must be emotionally faced and acknowledged by you, before it can be rightly met or filled by me. The real issue, the fear of my not coming through for you, and the lie the enemy has whispered to all of my children – that this struggle will never end – has to surface from where it has been buried in your heart. This is necessary in order for you to be able to fully meet me as the Prince of Peace in these present circumstances. Adversity breaks through the facade of your life and exposes the way you wrongly believed you had to have your life work in order to feel safe and fulfilled. Adversity strips you down to bear bones and brings you face to face with your neediness. This is where you will find real intimacy with me – by entering your own neediness. Neediness comes from hunger. You were created with hunger, it has just been twisted through the Fall of man. It can now become part of my redemption plan for you when you finally become willing to stop running, burying, or trying to fill it with other things."*

"Remain in me and I will remain in you and together we will walk each day in the surprises of the day. And yes, there will be many joys and releases to be found in each day as you give up the ways that seem right to you and receive and walk in the ways I have prepared for you. Surrender to me." "Remain in me, and I will remain in you. No branch can bear fruit by itself; it must remain in the vine. Neither can you bear fruit unless you remain in me." (John 15:4)

My Struggle:

Father, I'm confused about which way to go. I've asked and asked, but you have seemingly not answered yet. How long O Lord – Please direct my paths, I feel like nothing is happening...

God's Response to Me:

"My child, come, come with me, I am here. I desire to bring you even higher in your walk with me. You are trying to run ahead before you have even been prepared for that next step. I know you think you need to move ahead, but I want to lead you on the HIGHway of Isaiah 35. Wait for me to lead, you must not run ahead... that is the impulsiveness of a child not yet trained. I always move in the fullness of my time which is the perfect time prepared for you. We must walk together, be yoked together, and if you will remain internally just tucked in under my wing, you will experience rest. Remember, no matter whatever is or isn't happening... I AM. I AM your safe place of rest, your true security, your only real security, and I will surely lead you into your next step... Wait for me. Come, rest in me."
Matthew 11:28-30, Ps 23, Jeremiah 29:11

From the devotional Jesus Calling, January 15, *"The closer you live to Me, the safer you are. Circumstances around you are undulating and there are treacherous-looking waves in the distance. Fix your eyes on Me, the One who never changes. By the time those waves reach you, they will have shrunk to proportions of My design. I am always beside you, helping you face today's waves. The future is a phantom, seeking to spook you. Laugh at the future! Stay close to Me."*

CHAPTER 4
Reconciliation, Redemption, Restoration

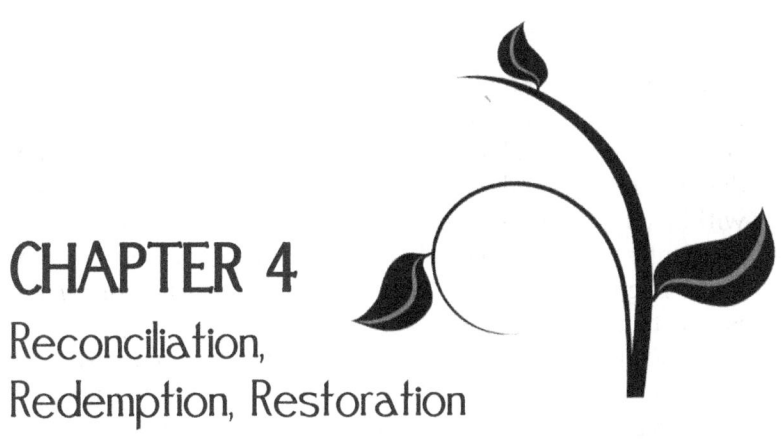

Many of us who make up the older generation were originally taught that the Christian life was about doing ministry, having a testimony of words, and witnessing to people about the gospel. Unfortunately, although those things are important, they often became a way of doing, a way of performing, a way of getting identity and worth, and feeling like "a good Christian". Too often those good things came from outside of our deepest selves, not from a changed life and character on the inside as Jesus said was necessary (Matthew 23:26). We became *human doings* instead of *human beings* with the life of God flowing through, but sadly we never knew there was another way.

Because of God's mercy, many good things still came from that approach and most of us walked in all we understood at the time. However a quick glance at the fruit that often came forth from that view of Christianity revealed the downfall of many of those ministries. Far too often included in that paradigm, was the *use* of other people to build their own ministries, mishandled finances, control and abuses of all kinds that caused both the world and much of the church to become disillusioned. Too much of it was about us – and our getting worth from it, not about God and co-laboring with him in his ways. *"All a man's ways seem innocent to him, but motives are weighed by The Lord."* (Proverbs 16:2)

However, as we finally began to allow the Spirit of God to search our hearts, shake loose the systems we had built to survive, and reveal the motivations of our hearts, a new desperately dependent way of living from the life of Jesus within us began to take its place. When we allow him to dismantle our old survival systems, a new starting place of *doing* begins to grow out of our *being in him*. Then our *living* is able to eventually come more and more from his life inside of us. From that starting place, what we do emanates from the center of our being where Jesus dwells. As a result, the Spirit is able to bring forth rivers of *his* living water to others through the unique gifts he has placed within us.

At the same time we find the world teaching that real life is about being successful, looked up to, admired, esteemed, and self-satisfied. The younger generation and the message of self they are bombarded with continually; whether through social media, advertisements, internet, *movies, or TV, life becomes very selfishly, totally about me.* Then the focus of life becomes – *"How can I get what I want?" "What brings me pleasure?" "What appears to momentarily satisfy the tremendous hole in my heart?"* There is a season on the healing journey however, that by outward appearances might look to be selfish, but is really a time of learning with Jesus how to re-nurture the empty places within. It is joining with him in self-nurturing the areas that have gotten trampled, abused, forgotten, abandoned, and lost. More on that subject can be found in my last book, <u>Born to Fly</u>.

Under the searching in all the wrong places for satisfaction is a God-given longing to be seen, known, valued, and accepted with all of the good, bad, and ugly that still lurks within all of us. The hidden cry of our souls is for someone to really *see* us, *hear* us, someone to please *accept* us, and *value* us. In the original creation, we were meant to be seen, known, heard, accepted, and valued, but that was lost through the Fall. In its place man experienced the fear of shame and failure and was terrified of being found out as not having what it takes. A competition began that drove man to be seen and valued through his performance in any area that he deemed important. He worked on developing the gifts or desires that suited him and brought him the strokes he was longing to experience.

What would give him the worth he desired? Perhaps a relationship in which he/she felt pursued, children who made him/her feel needed, a career where he/she was recognized and admired, money that he believed would bring freedom, things to fill the hole inside, a ministry in which he/she was looked up to, or a sports performance where cheered and celebrated? What might yours be? Mine: I had sadly used people and ministry.

"Come, all you are thirsty, come to the waters; and you who have no money, come buy and eat. Come, buy wine and milk without money and without cost. Why spend money on what is not bread and your labor on what does not satisfy? Listen, listen to me and eat what is good, and your soul will delight in the richest of fare. Give ear and come to me; hear me, that your soul may live..." (Isaiah 55:1,2)

Because we don't feel much value and worth inside ourselves, we look for it outside of us. We too often settle for admiration when we really longing to be loved. Ask yourself the question – *"Do I really desire to be loved or admired?"* Admiration is cold, detached, enjoyed from afar, and it still leaves us disconnected from what we are really desiring on a heart level. Like a valuable piece of art in a museum, you can admire it, but not have a relationship with it. Love warms the heart. The longing deep inside us is to be loved, known as we really are with all our flaws and still be accepted. We desire to be valued, not judged as unworthy and then dismissed. Too much of our society has a throw-away mentality, a spirit of dismissal. It looks something like this: *"If you please me by doing what I want, I will keep you around, however, when you displease me, I will replace you with someone who is more acceptable to me!"*

The Atmosphere We Carry and the "Name" It Gives Us

Someone I will refer to as Jeff, was rejected by his father and left hungry for male acceptance. Nurture comes from the mother, but because masculinity is bestowed by masculinity, when a father doesn't "name" his son with eyes of love and acceptance that see the boy's uniqueness and value that, the son receives a "name" from the atmosphere that the father projects. Sometimes the naming comes with horrible words, like stupid, failure, or something similar. However, it can also be a naming of shame even though words of that nature were never spoken; perhaps just a disgruntled look or a sigh that speaks volumes! It is also possible that because a father figure was absent in the boy's life, he was left nameless so he has never been able to see himself as valuable, as having what it takes. God's desire to re-father us all in a concrete way becomes possible once we have faced our pain and unearthed the lies of shame that have named us.

We all carry an atmosphere whether we are aware of it or not. Whenever we enter a room, we carry an atmosphere that will either draw in, invite, or instead close out, and push away. I have people tell me all the time that nobody likes them, accepts them or even speaks to them when they enter a room. A closer look reveals they are carrying a shut-down atmosphere to which people are simply responding. The atmosphere we experienced in our original families might have been accepting, rejecting, or maybe even indifferent. When it is a healthy atmosphere, you feel welcomed and enjoyed and learn to see and accept yourself as enjoyable.

That healthy atmosphere of a home carries with it a message that you are valuable and worth getting to know even if you are a bit different from their picture of how they think you should be. If unhealthy, it reveals to you the opposite, that you are to be judged as insignificant and not worth knowing or accepting on any deep level. Even the indifference gives us a name that causes us to feel ignored, erased, or invisible, not really worth seeing, and it shuts us down. The message the child longs to receive though is that you believe they have what it takes, that you really see and accept them, that they are valuable to you just the way they are – not after they have been remade into your own image for them.

Many parents who have never dealt with their own rejection issues, interpret as rejection what is simply the behavior of a child who is in emotional pain or confused by their own emotions. Sadly that parent reacts to their child with rejection because they mistakenly feel the child is rejecting them. In that case, the parent is unfortunately acting out of the woundedness of the rejected little child who is still hidden inside themselves. That gives even more reason for allowing the Spirit of God to search us and heal our own broken hearts because we can only give to our children what we have gotten for ourselves. Once again we must hear the message the flight attendant gives at the beginning of every flight, to put the oxygen mask on yourself before you attempt to put it on your child. That spiel always seemed wrong to me, but the truth is we can only give another that which we truly have for ourselves. Many parents try to do the opposite of what their parents did, yet it still comes out of their own woundedness and often simply does harm in a different way.

The Atmosphere of a Home

The atmosphere we carry can penetrate our home by giving forth a message of performance and perfectionism. Your home can be admired by those who visit, but is it welcoming?

CHAPTER 4

Do people feel free to relax, kick back and enjoy or is it just a beautiful dwelling? The Bible speaks of hospitality, but that is not just something we do. We can give forth an image of hospitality with all the best foods, beautiful surroundings and yet still have that simply be worldly entertaining. True hospitality is a spirit we release from within us that is welcoming, and the setting has little to do with it. Being in the most humble abode with only a glass of cold water, can feel more warm and inviting than entering a palatial mansion with a feast set before you.

Jill was forced to move from a lovely house because of some very difficult circumstances. Her former home was truly a place where her gracious gift of hospitality was easily released. The nice rental house Jill moved into was much smaller and to her, uninviting. Since her circumstances were not going to change anytime soon, she was forced to grieve the loss of her former home. As she did, Jill began to see her new little abode in a very different light and finally became ready to make it her home. Now the spirit of hospitality Jill carries will be released there, just as it was in her former home, because it's not in the house, but within herself.

With all the houses on television that are showcased, it's easy to become lured into the image or illusion of desiring a gorgeous home like that. Unfortunately, what far too often is created, is a place that doesn't really feel like a home that is warm and welcoming – beautiful, yes, but not inviting. There is a huge difference between a spectacular house that you want to drool over and a humble place of acceptance and rest. I am also amazed at some of the reality television shows dealing with the extremely dysfunctional, out of control families who live in a gorgeous houses. In that case obviously much time and money has gone into the decorating, but little into creating a warm atmosphere of acceptance and delight.

As a teenager, I wanted to be anywhere but at my own house. I call it a house because that's what it was – it never felt like a home. I always felt on the outside looking in so when I finally got my own wheels, many evenings I drove around late into the night just to delay having to go home. How sad when a child doesn't feel any loving warmth in their own home – unfortunately we see far too many teens finding a "family" with their peers and looking for any place else to be where they feel welcomed. I sadly know of a teen who even wanted to join a gang for that reason. He was continually ridiculed, verbally abused, and totally unaccepted in his own family, so to him, a gang meant people who were looking out for him. He felt a sense of "family" and belonging.

That is why it's important to see that the atmosphere we create is of great importance even from the time our children are babies. Babies and young children can absorb the atmosphere of a home that does not have a welcoming, secure feeling, and react to it, though of course they have no intellectual capacity to understand so as to put it into words. Parents who have unhealed animosity toward each other, even when it's seemingly held underground, can release a rejecting, insecure atmosphere in their home for their children.

One strange way this lack of warmth and acceptance can play out is this – I have had a number of adults tell me about their children's anger that causes the child to act out in inappropriate ways. Young children can act out very irresponsibly when they feel emotional pain or insecurity simply because they don't know what to do with what they are feeling. One of those ways is sometimes to react badly to the one they feel is the source of their pain. Or in some cases even to reject the one who is the safest person in their household while accepting the one who is more abusive. In that case, anger at the abusive parent can be displaced by putting it on the one who feels safer. Children often act out of confused feelings. It would be far too dangerous to reject the one who feels more threatening, but much easier to let it out on the safe parent. It doesn't make logical sense, but unhealed feelings don't make logical sense, they are emotions.

My husband, who was extremely logical, used to get frustrated with various people because their behavior didn't make sense! I reminded him over and over not to expect an emotionally-driven, wounded person to make sense – they can't, they are often acting out of a much earlier age in their lives where the unhealed emotions still remain. When triggered, that person reverts back to three or four years old, or wherever the pain is still lodged.

Renaming

There are often unspoken words, maybe only coming from attitude or body language, that can emanate from the parent to the child that imply, *"What's wrong with you?"* Or the child is sometimes spoken to with a shaming, angry tone of voice even though there are no specific shaming words. Some of the most painful "words" we have heard are those not spoken aloud, but still communicated through a disgusted sigh or even silence – however, they *"named"* that child just the same. One parent told me they were careful only to speak positively to their child. Yes, the words were positive, but the presentation was demeaning. The child was still named as not enough, not measuring up, not worth it, a failure.

My own father named me through his incessant teasing which contained disguised put-downs. Teasing from my father and shaming judgments from my mother caused me to believe I was really ugly and deformed. Words spoken with either disdain or mocking laughter like, "your hair is too straight, you have a pug nose like a fighter, your neck is too bony, you are too skinny" all communicated to me as a developing young girl that I was unacceptable – there was something very wrong with me. I was even told by my mother that I shouldn't ever wear the color purple because it looked so bad on me. Yet much to my surprise, many years later when I was finally becoming me, I discovered that purple was one of my best colors! It was my mother's judgment and rejection of herself that she put on me, and I carried it for years as shame over myself. It was really her shame, not mine. The greatest gift we can give our children is to get healthy ourselves.

For so many, their hidden heart cry is, *"Does anyone see me as having value?"* They have been told, whether with or without words that they don't measure up to the standard, whatever that standard might be. They are bringing their question of who they are to others, but because the others have been wounded as well, they cannot answer their question or they answer it wrongly with an *implied, "No, you don't measure up"*. It is dangerous to bring ourselves to others to find our worth because then the people, whoever they might be, rule and determine who we are. No, we must first face our question and then bring it to God to discover who it was he created before we ever stepped foot into this broken world.

In 1 Samuel 15, we find that King Saul was rejected from being king because he *"was small in his own eyes"* and so allowed the people to rule instead of getting his direction from God and walking in obedience as King David did. He feared the people and needed their acceptance so they ended up ruling. Whenever we are walking in the fear of man, we are doing the same thing and allowing the people to rule us, whoever our "significant people" happen to be.

One woman, I will call Erica, was always looking for validation from her husband. Unfortunately though, her husband had experienced false naming through the rejection he felt from his own father and the ongoing control, containing a hidden message from his mother implying, *"You don't have what it takes so I have to tell you what to do"*. As a result, he was unable to even see his wife's worth, no less name her as precious to him. The more she tried to *pull* acceptance from him, the more he pulled away, rejecting her advances with whatever things would help to fill the emptiness in his own heart. He used things like validation in his career, the recognition he got from the things he did well like golf, and the seeking of all kinds of pleasure, most of which never included her. Unfortunately, she was trying to get her husband to illegitimately name her in order to fill the empty hole in her heart left from never being named as valuable from her own family. In that case both had been wrongly named by their parents and each was seeking to find their worth from the wrong sources.

Psalm 139:14 names us as *"fearfully and wonderfully made"*. Since God knew us before our parents met us for the first time, he is the only one who can rightly name us! *"O Lord, you have searched me and you know me."* (Psalm 139:1) *"...Before I was born The Lord called me; from my birth he has made mention of my name."* (Isaiah 49:1b) God knew us and called us prior to our parents giving any name to us! God named us first – before any of the robbery of a broken world happened to us! He alone has the original blueprint for our lives.

God, as a Father, named Jesus as he was beginning his public ministry before all the people when he said, *"This is my Son, whom I love; with him I am well pleased"*. (Matthew 3:17) He named Jesus again on the Mount of Transfiguration when he spoke from heaven, *"This is my Son, whom I love; with him I am well pleased. Listen to him!"* (Matthew 17:5) God desires to rename us as well, and because of Jesus' sacrifice, renaming is possible if we will shed the name we have been given through shame, even if it was just implied. That can't be only done intellectually however, we must face the pain and the shame of self it caused us by wrongly naming us. It is the *shame name* we must release, coming out of agreement with it, and then being willing to come to Jesus who came to heal the brokenhearted, and who longs to bestow on us new name. *"...You will be called by a new name that the mouth of The Lord will bestow. You will be a crown of splendor in the*

Lord's hand, a royal diadem in the hand of your God. No longer will they call you Deserted or name your land Desolate... for The Lord will take delight in you..." (Isaiah 62:2-4)

Real or Legitimate Shame

My question to you: Will you discover and release your old name and receive the name prepared for you from the foundation of the world? (Ephesians 1:4-6). In order to do that, we must recognize the difference between real shame and false shame. We all have real shame when we sin and come short of God's standard. Every person who ever lived after the fall, except for Jesus, has had legitimate or real shame. None of us has measured up and that's one of the reasons, Jesus the only perfect person, had to sacrifice his life for us. *"For all have sinned and fall short of the glory of God."* (Romans 3:23) *"We all, like sheep, have gone astray, each one of us has turned to his own way; and The Lord has laid on him the iniquity of us all."* (Isaiah 53:6)

The beauty of the cross is that when we come to him, he offers us forgiveness and acceptance – just as if we'd never sinned. *"If we confess our sins, he is faithful and just and will forgive us our sins and purify us from all unrighteousness."* (1 John 1:9). Psalm 32 tells us the same. If we do not push our sin under the carpet or beat ourselves up for it, but simply own it and bring it to the cross, he is there waiting for us with great desire to forgive, cleanse, and release us from all guilt! Jesus has prepared a table for us with a warm welcome to take our place at his table, to sit in the chair he pulls out for us, the chair that no one else can sit in. Even if we refuse it – it's still ours, waiting for us.

False or Illegitimate Shame and a Shame-Based Identity

However, mixed with our real shame is often a false shame, one that is not ours legitimately. That shame does not come from something we did. It was the shame of another person that was put on us through their words, false guilting, or actions, and is not legitimately ours – it belongs to that person. Abuse is an example of false shaming whether it be emotional, verbal, mental, physical, or sexual. Sadly, when a child is abused in any way, even through peers in the neighborhood growing up, it damages the identity of the child and gives them a false way of seeing themselves. Instead of being able to love and accept themselves, they view themselves through the eyes of the shame that actually belongs to another. We are never meant to carry someone else's shame!

Adults are meant to protect children, care for them, but instead when a child is harmed through abuse of any kind, even what we might consider minor abuse, the child feels dirty, not valuable and a lie is formed at the deepest core of their being. The lie has different words for different people, but generally the feeling is similar in its essence. The shame of the lie is, *"I'm not worth anything!"* Sadly, the child often feels shame for even the desire to be wanted and enjoyed. That desire to be loved and protected is a God-given longing we are all born with and one that is good, not bad. However, as a result of the abuse or bad treatment, their longings now feel wrong and the child begins to hate even their desires. As an unfortunate consequence of that self-rejection, the child begins to abandon the deepest part of their heart and create a false self just to survive. That false self might include being a performer, perfectionist, clown, pleaser, or it could reveal itself in an angry, rebellious persona that hates and continually sabotages itself.

Any false shame we are carrying for another person must be recognized as theirs and separated from any of our own legitimate shame. Once separated, it can be given back to whomever it belongs. You do not do it verbally to the person, but it can be most helpful to make a list of everything you feel shame over, and separate it out. Separate the real shame from any of the false shame you might be carrying for someone else and refuse to carry it for them any longer.

A shame lie about ourselves might also have come in through the atmosphere of our home. I was born into an atmosphere of shame in my home and so it was absorbed from the beginning. Shaming could have also happened to us in school or through teachers or other authority figures – even something significant that happened with our peers. That false shame belief might be the result of unhealed feelings of rejection or abandonment by key people in our lives, or through various failures we experienced embarrassment over.

Discovering God's Truth About Us

Failure is only shame if we refuse to learn from it. Those false shame beliefs must be recognized and released as the lies they are. *Who are we really?* Only God can reveal that to our hearts as we seek his opinion and begin to accept the truth of his Word. The hole left in our hearts from the removal of the lie then needs to be replaced with God's truth about us. Psalm 51 reminds us that the truth God desires for us is not in our minds alone, but in our innermost being, deep within our hearts. That takes our active participation with him in the process of releasing the lie of our shame and then becoming willing to forgive those who have falsely named us.

We have to then rename ourselves with the name God offers to us. If we have carried a shame message through how we have been named in our original family, he offers us *his name* to replace it. Let me give you an example from my own life. I had always hated my name and everything else about myself when I was trapped by a shame identity. One day God led me to look up the name Patricia and I learned it meant "honorable family". My first thought was, "That's far from the truth!". Then God quietly spoke to my heart, *"I adopted you into my family and now you carry my family name"*. That family is honorable! As we begin to allow ourselves to be re-identified, we bring ourselves to others as enjoyable and worth knowing, instead of looking to others to tell us whether we are valuable or not. We teach them how to treat us simply by the way we see, respect, and enjoy ourselves. We then give the power of naming us back to the Source of *true life* instead of to others who are simply wounded themselves.

I encourage you to look again at the atmosphere or presence you carry – is it one of openness with the invitation for others to enjoy you, or is it one of holding back and hiding your true self? Might you be trying to get your life and acceptance from others, or from what you do? Do you wear a mask because you have viewed your real self as unacceptable? Look at the atmosphere of the home you grew up in as well as your home now – is it a safe one where it is acceptable for a person to be who they are without abusive criticism or without fearing the withholding of your love? Observe the atmosphere that others bring with them as well, not in judgment, but in order to try to draw them out, praying for their release too. God longs for us to participate with him in providing a welcoming atmosphere for those he brings into our lives.

For many, it is easier to be open and vulnerable with people outside of our family than it is with those inside our own home. We are often afraid of openness and vulnerability at home because they are the ones with the ability to most hurt us. And yet the first people we must release an atmosphere of open love to are those in our closest circle. For too many years the church has wanted to run to the far corners of the earth to pour out their love while those closest to them felt rejected and abandoned. For a number of years now, the Lord has reminded me of his pattern from Acts 1:8b, *"...you will be my witnesses in Jerusalem, Judea, Samaria, and to the ends of the earth"*. Notice that being a witness (not preaching, but *being*) begins in our own Jerusalem. For Jesus Jerusalem was a place of death and resurrection, and so it is for us. We must be willing to die to self and our own self-protection, which is the opposite of love, at home instead of escaping home to run to the ends of the earth. It's then from our Jerusalem we go forth in resurrection life!

CHAPTER 5
Grieving Our Disappointed Desires and Losses

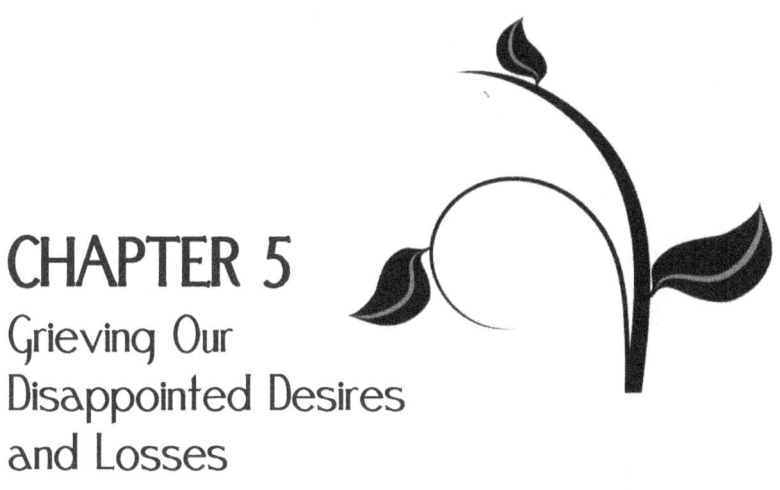

If we begin to allow ourselves to view life without our rose colored glasses, we often come face to face with some disappointed desires, frustrations, injustices, and a general reflection of the brokenness of the world we live in that we have spent a lifetime trying to push away or control. However the more we allow ourselves to face that reality, we begin to see with new eyes of wonder that the difficult and sad are often mixed in with the beautiful and wonderful. In the same hour we can experience a wonderful "gift" through a moment of joy along with a "major disappointed desire". How do we handle that mixture? Remember, we all desire to live "happily ever after" as the fairy tales have portrayed it for us. That would have been our experience had we remained in the Garden, but unfortunately the Fall of Man in the Garden of Eden destroyed that picture completely.

Many of us have spent far too much energy trying to recreate the perfection of the Garden in this world the way it was originally intended to be. In that struggle, we often find ourselves angry, frustrated, depressed, and struggling to make life work according to our picture, and to make it be fair. The reality is that this world isn't fair – it wasn't fair for Jesus as they abused him and hung him on a cross even though he was the only perfect person who had ever lived! If it wasn't fair for Jesus, you can bet it won't be fair at times in our own lives. Having our eyes opened to see the many gifts God is giving, some very small and others that are amazingly huge, right along with the losses of our lives, brings new adventure to each day. And living without trying to control our circumstances allows God to flow through our lives in wonderful ways! As we become willing to cooperate with him, he frees us to live in a new place of peace even in the midst of the storms of life.

What do we do with the fears that trigger the insecurities of life? What about the desires for those things our hearts were created for, things for which we had hope? What do we do with that slow ache that resides far down in the depths of our soul, the vague feelings of disillusionment that we have experienced, but have avoided over and over. Those disappointments might be revealed in a special relationship, job, church, and even with God, or ourselves. We don't always notice our ache as long as we can stay busy enough and hide those feelings under the survival systems we have created. If we are to keep our hearts alive and face our disappointments, we must be able to do something with that ache, so finding God's way of dealing with our disappointed and thwarted desires is a must.

Releasing Our Losses Through Grief

God's way of helping us to release the losses of any kind is through grieving. Too often we put grieving only in the category of death, but it is far bigger than that. Any loss, major or seemingly minor, when mourned, can be released. Grieving begins with acknowledgment by facing the pain of our loss, not just in general, but as our particular loss. It is giving value to the voice of our own heart in that moment by listening to what our heart is speaking to us even though difficult. Because our emotions are the voice of our hearts, they are telling us what our heart is feeling in that moment. If we refuse to listen, we can stay stuck in that particular emotion of grief for years even though we bury it and try to move on.

I can give you an example of that with someone I have met with. Rachel had a similar dream over and over through the years, always having to do with the house in which she grew up. She always awoke feeling fearful and uneasy and began to have a dread of those dreams. As she began to face some of the pain she felt in her childhood and grieve some of the losses she experienced, the dreams lessened. Recently she revealed she hasn't had one now for several years! It's not uncommon for unhealed emotions and unshed grief to come out in our dreams.

Carrie had been stuck in grief for most of her life and didn't know it. It began with the rejections and losses from her dad in early childhood, then repeated over and over through sports, relationships, jobs, even ministry. She was stuck in blame and as long as she continued to blame those who had failed her, Carrie wasn't able to mourn her losses and truly release them. By holding onto her resentments, she was sadly setting herself up for more failure and rejection, and sabotaging herself in relationship after relationship through the un-faced grief she was carrying within. She remained a very angry person. Finally after far too many years went by, and after she became so miserable in her life, Carrie began to realize she needed to face the pain of the rejections and enter her grief. Finally after releasing her losses to Jesus, she allowed him to heal her broken heart and was eventually able to forgive all those who had harmed her.

Ancient Israel knew much more about grieving than we seem to understand. They would call for the wailing women to help facilitate the grief process, but we just try to get over it! The map at the Mall that gives you your present location with the message, "You Are Here" helps you to get to your

CHAPTER 5

destination. In the same way, as a person finally ceases to deny that they are in an emotional struggle, then they are ready. They feel the pain yes, but it also brings release and the beginning of healing as they allow themselves to finally grieve and release their losses.

There is a difference between grieving and mourning in that a person can be trapped in their grief for years, but never release it by mourning. Mourning requires recognizing specifically what you are grieving and then allowing the sorrow to work its way through to final acceptance. As I grieved my husband's death, it was necessary for me to know specifically what I was mourning each time a new wave of grief would hit. As soon as I recognized the specifics, like, "I will always come home to an empty house now" or "I no longer have someone to do things with", and face the loss, I would pass through the sorrow and enter a new place of peace, and then as time went on, joy.

One woman I meet with has suffered a number of losses in her original family; as well as a job loss with many resulting financial insecurities, a child leaving home for the first time, and a major health issue. These all happened pretty much in the same time period. Combined, they left her feeling more and more overwhelmed and unglued. Cyndi began to freak out even more as she became increasingly undone and thought she was losing it! Through what was happening, she was forced to face some major fears concerning the loss of security in key areas of her life. There were issues Cyndi had to struggle out with God, such as, Was he enough to keep her from destruction? He certainly wasn't doing things according to her picture of how he was supposed to act. By finally being willing to be totally honest about her feelings with God, Cyndi eventually, with much fear and trembling, came to a new place of surrender to his loving care and peace. As I suggested she might also be mourning her picture of how she thought life would look for her, she resonated with it and recognized she was grieving a broken picture of life, and even of God!

"...Weeping may remain for a night, but rejoicing comes in the morning." (Psalm 30:5b)

"You turned my wailing into dancing; you removed my sackcloth and clothed me with joy." (Psalm 30:11)

My Own Journey of Grief

I would like to share with you my own personal journey of grieving, with its many struggles and feelings in the hopes that it will aid you in grieving any losses of your own. These losses often go unrecognized, and yet can affect our lives in some of the various ways I will share below. Often without realizing it, our un-faced losses can cause us to remain stuck and unable to move forward. Far too often, they go way back into our childhood, or young adult years, and at other times they are the result of the circumstances we are presently struggling with.

A woman I once worked with had lost her husband five years before I met her. She had never allowed herself to mourn and instead completely buried herself with work. I knew there was something wrong when I saw how driven she was to work and accomplish things, even becoming demanding of the others she worked with to do the same. It didn't help that she was the boss! As a result, no one liked to work with her, but when we talked, I realized she had never finished grieving her husband's death. As we opened up that floodgate, she began to face the things she should have grieved five years earlier and finally allowed herself to mourn. At long last, she was able to finally go on with her real life much more peacefully for everyone. Grief doesn't go away, it simply goes underground if it is not shed.

CHAPTER 5

Some of the many ways those un-grieved losses may have affected us could include our health, both physical and emotional, or even sleep patterns with a desire to sleep too much or on the other side, the inability to get to sleep and stay asleep. The un-grieved losses might also have caused old fears to surface, be experienced as a general sense of anxiety or out of control feelings, and perhaps even an inability to concentrate. One person I know would fall asleep whenever the pain seeped in. In some, it can cause the drive to escape or avoid through various means like, work, alcohol, meds, depression, etc. There is certainly nothing wrong with needed medication as long as the under-lying issues are being addressed as well. Un-faced grief can also cause feelings of being continually fatigued, bored, overwhelmed with the simplest of tasks, distraction to the point of feeling you are losing your memory, confused, and left with a feeling that nothing you do ever satisfies. You can also be left with an emptiness, feeling like you have a hole in your heart, or a hopelessness that nothing seems to reach. On the other hand, the anger connected to that loss can cause you to become a blamer of others because they are not meeting your needs.

Since we all walk through our grief in a very personal way, it's important to recognize the symptoms that are common to our own particular grief since they can vary with different people. My most common grief symptom is distraction and the inability to think clearly. I might be driving to a specific destination and without any awareness, begin to drive in the wrong direction even though I am totally familiar with the way to go and may have done it countless times. When that begins to happen, it has now become a warning that I'm grieving something I am unconsciously ignoring. A friend recently went to the wrong airport to pick up a family member simply because she had so much on her mind that she was pushing aside instead of taking the needed time to work it through.

I just recently recognized another symptom of my personal grieving – that symptom comes out in my body as pain in my left hip. For three months after my husband died, I lived with a chronic ache that began right after his death in that left hip. As we tend to do, I blamed it on my mattress! As my grieving began to subside a bit, so did the pain. Recently, as I was grieving a loss over a family situation, I awoke with the same pain in my left hip. I hadn't experienced it for, almost two years, but as I became aware it was a symptom of my grief and allowed myself to write about what I was feeling with the current loss, my pain let up quite a bit. However, because the pain caused me to limp for quite a while, several more steps were necessary to see it fully healed. In the future, I will be much more aware that it might be a warning sign to me that I have some unshed loss to face.

Not everyone experiences all of the symptoms or even experiences them in the same way. So if you are not experiencing them all or perhaps you might even have different ones, do not necessarily discount the fact you might be grieving, particularly if there has been a major, or even what you have dismissed as a minor loss of some kind in your life, either past or present. Of course some of those symptoms can also come from other things, so I encourage you to ask God to reveal if you might be grieving. When we are grieving, becoming aware of it can be a blessing and a way through to the other side. So what do we do with grief? We own it, feel it, name it, connect it to the circumstance, and eventually come through to a new place of release and joy. Jesus, the man of sorrows, grieves with us when we invite him.

Even though grieving is a very personal experience, there are common stages we all go through in one way or another. How deeply we experience the feelings and how long the process takes will depend on the nature of the grief and the person's own make-up, as well as if there is significant grief from the past that has never been faced.

For example, let's say you experienced a painful betrayal earlier in life that was never grieved all the way through. Then a situation happens at work where you experience a betrayal of trust from a co-worker you had previously trusted. That current experience can reopen the old wound and cause you an inability to forgive and move on in the present. I call that a set-up. Our strong reaction to the present situation and our inability to get past it, sets us up to recognize there might be a previous loss we have never grieved.

Grief is a painful part of the fallen, broken world we find ourselves living in. In good times we can almost pretend there is no sorrow that has to be faced and grieved, but then something like some of the earlier examples or another type of loss affects us that proves otherwise. We all long to live happily ever after – no wonder romantic movies are so popular and perhaps why we were so drawn to the fairy tales, daydreaming, fantasy, or science fiction movies as children. Without even realizing it, we might be still choosing fantasy or magical thinking instead of facing the painful realities of life. Unconsciously, many do that even with God and then feel depressed when he doesn't perform as they would have liked.

A world of our own creation is so much prettier and far more perfect than the reality of the broken world we currently find ourselves living in. We all have disappointed desires... things we hoped for that never happened. Perhaps it was a relationship, a career, ministry, or you even might have feelings of being deserted by loved ones in your time of need, or even by God. These are the things that must be faced and grieved so we can go on with real living that comes from our hearts instead of just pretending and getting by.

Losses

Life has a way of happening to us all at one time or another. Some painful loss breaks into the satisfactory life we have created for ourselves and we are thrown into a sometimes frightening unknown season. It could be a season of deeper loss than any we might have walked through before, such as the death of a loved one, as I experienced this past season with the loss of my husband of over 50 plus years.

It could concern the loss of an income, a career, a house, a relationship or even the loss of hope for something prayed for over a long period with no change. It might have been the loss of a place in which you felt valued and needed, or even the loss of a beloved pet. It could be the loss of our particular "picture" of the way we believed our life should have looked by now. When our picture shatters through circumstances, we get undone. The chaotic world we are presently living in has broken through the false realities for many, even affecting what was known as the American dream. Look at the shattered pictures of so many Americans when the housing crisis struck our nation. For so many, their picture of having it all was destroyed.

We all long for a world without pain and heartbreak, and one day, if our life has been given over to Jesus, we will experience that life. Thankfully, my husband is tasting it now. Wonderful for him to be free of his suffering, but sad for me with the loss of his presence on a day to day basis. What do we do with losses such as these? Do we just try to suck it up and go on? Our feelings of loss have to be felt in our emotions and then further faced by looking at any false beliefs we had about how life should work for us.

(Hebrews 11:16) *"...they were longing for a better country – a heavenly one. Therefore God is not ashamed to be called their God for he has prepared a city for them."*

Our silent demands and false beliefs have to be looked at, grieved, released to God, and then finally replaced with the truth from God's Word. As we do that, we can begin to view life from God's perspective and discover an even greater measure of security that originates from God's eternal truth. When we honestly face our fears and losses, then are willing to struggle through them with God, there can be a birthing of a new security that begins to develop right in the midst of the losses and troubles we are experiencing – a strange peace that passes understanding. That peace comes from finally discovering there is someone greater than our circumstances walking with us. We are not alone.

There are stages to grief and going through them is a process we have to enter instead of trying to avoid. Depending on the grief material you read, the descriptions tend to vary a bit, but generally they include: Shock - Denial - Feelings of Betrayal - Bargaining with God - Anger, Disappointment - Sorrow - Acceptance.

To walk through the process, however long it takes, requires feeling our own disappointed desires and losses, our anger, sadness, powerlessness, and uncertainty for the future. In the midst of that, the enemy usually lies and taunts us about our future, to the tune of something like, *"You know things will never change. You will be trapped in this pain of loss forever."* It is imperative we recognize that taunt as the lie it is and not agree with it.

Our own plans haven't worked, so we are then forced to learn to trust God in new ways with our future. It is in the midst of the struggle of feeling those disappointed emotions that we must meet Jesus who suffered every emotion we do and whose mission was, and still is, to *"heal our broken hearts"* (Isaiah 61). He is already in our future and his plans are good, but the degree of our anger or anxiety reveals how little we are believing that with our hearts – in our minds maybe, but not in the depths of our hearts. *"As a man thinketh in his heart so is he"*. (Proverbs 23:7 KJV)

A very human tendency is for us either to feel trapped in our emotions or to choose to bury the overwhelmed and out of control feelings. When we do, the feelings often come out by trying to try to control lesser things. Whenever a person begins to exhibit control by trying to line their ducks up in the smaller things, there is often a much larger area in which they are feeling out of control. For example, let's say there is a major problem on the job and you are feeling fearful and powerless, or your teen seems distant and rebellious, or you have health issues you can't resolve. It's not uncommon then to find yourself trying to control the little things within the home that really don't matter and then get angry when everyone else doesn't cooperate!

Some people shut down completely, others get even busier to cover the pain of loss like the woman I mentioned earlier who hid herself in work. We try to use anything that seems to work to cover and avoid the emptiness, sorrow, disappointment, powerlessness, fear, anxiety, and anger. Unfortunately though, in order to keep from feeling the struggle within us, we must avoid and deaden our own hearts. Our hearts are the very place the Bible tells us we must live from if we are to be truly alive and present in our own lives and move into our future with joy. Interestingly, real joy comes through facing our sorrows. That joy is far greater than the happiness that is derived just from good "happenings".

Because I desire not to only present the grieving journey in a clinical way, below I am sharing my own personal, struggle with the various feelings of grief in a very up-close and personal way. My desire is that you might find it helpful on your particular journey. Even though each person is unique in their own expression, there are also feelings that are common to man. But first let's look more closely at the various symptoms of grief.

Common Symptoms of Grief:

- Tightness or heaviness in the throat or chest
- Denial of the reality of the grief
- Restlessness
- Inability to concentrate, Distraction
- Anger at God or the loved one
- Unexpected crying or other emotion, waves of sadness, disappointed desires
- Physical weakness
- Difficulty with sleep, dreams of the loved one
- Forgetfulness and struggle with memory
- Loss of appetite
- Feeling empty, forsaken, all alone
- Troubled by an inability to complete tasks
- Preoccupation with your loss
- Guilt feelings
- Feeling the need to caretake others' feelings and protecting them while neglecting your own

Those are just a few of the symptoms and you can see how they can affect our everyday lives. Grief tends to come in waves with periods of relative calm in between. At times though, the waves can be extremely intense and overwhelming. But as we begin to flow with them instead of pushing them away, they eventually begin to lose intensity and get farther apart. In the immediate months after my husband's death, I found myself doing quite well, actually better than I expected, but about six months after his death, a wave of intense grief hit me. I didn't realize at the time that its not uncommon to experience a fresh wave of grief like that sometimes even eight months later.

As the chronic illness my husband struggled with for years took a turn for the worse and became extremely serious, culminating in his death three weeks later, the over-riding emotion I experienced pretty much throughout, was peace. It was truly *"the peace that passes understanding"* and that peace continued to carry me through the days thereafter. In large part, that was because I had been grieving his impending death for many months prior to the actual event. I was aware this was an illness from which he would not recover because God had graciously prepared me that his time was approaching even before there were any serious symptoms.

However, another large contributing factor to my being able to walk in much peace in the aftermath, was that I had already grieved many other losses and disappointed longings throughout the years. As a result, the grief I experienced through his death was not added on top of the earlier losses, as it is for many. It is important to grieve each new loss as it comes so they do not accumulate and finally get triggered in an overwhelming way.

"And the peace of God which transcends all understanding, will guard your hearts and your minds in Christ Jesus." (Philippians 4:7)

One woman I meet with had never grieved her many earlier disappointed desires and struggles, so when a major loss hit through the unexpected ending of a job due to downsizing, she became intensely stuck in her grief and anger. She was unable move on with her life until she faced what she had previously buried. Terri had to sort out what she wrongly carried as her failure and shame, even when she had done nothing wrong, and recognize how the false shame she carried throughout her life was still affecting her.

It is not to say that in my personal struggle with grief after Bruce's death, I didn't struggle with many emotions – one

CHAPTER 5

particular emotion connected to my fear of my own inability and ineptness to do the things he had always handled with grace. It was downright scary, because I did make some mistakes in a few of the early decisions life forced me to make without him. In the past, we had never moved forward in any big decision without being in one accord so it always felt safe to trust the Lord's wisdom to come through one of us. Widespread good advice is that it is not helpful to make any life-changing decisions for at least a year after a major loss like death. Because of our grief, we are unclear on what is best for us even though we might think we know. I also felt very alone as I faced having to walk into my future without him, but for the most part, I experienced the overwhelming peace of God sustaining me. I was ok. Although there were times of distraction that allowed me to recognize another wave of grief was overtaking me, the peace never left, until...

Almost six months later, the intense wave of grief I mentioned earlier hit me! It came as a total surprise because I thought I was gradually healing. We never know all the aspects of grief until they get triggered by new circumstances. Upon looking up material on grieving, I found it not uncommon for a new wave of grief to come many months later causing mild depression and feelings of aloneness. It also comes at a time when others have less understanding because we seemed to be doing so well.

My new wave of grief was triggered by "firsts ". As summer approached, there was my birthday, Mother's Day, summer vacation, other holidays like Memorial Day, July 4th, a special family wedding and a grandson's graduation party... all firsts to be experienced *alone.*

Oh yes, I have a wonderful family that has truly been there for me. I couldn't ask for more in a caring, supportive family, but the first circle of family is with our spouse – the one with whom we enjoy things on a regular basis. The next circle is comprised of our adult children and their families who are each a family unto themselves, as it should be. As wonderful as it is when they include us in things, they are still their own family and there must be no *expectation* or *pull* put on them. The same with our friends, many have their own families and although we can have wonderful times of fellowship, we cannot *pull* on them to meet our needs either, but simply enjoy the gifts they are to us when those special times of connection come.

Part of my grieving process consisted of releasing the past connection with my spouse in the sense of having someone there to do things with, and then facing the unknown emptiness with God alone, and whatever family or friends he brought to me to share with at various times and in various ways. *Every good and perfect gift comes from above*, and on that new journey, we begin to know him in an even more intimate way. One such gift he brought to me in a totally unexpected way...

It is natural for widows to band together in the walking through the new season of aloneness. The problem was that at the time of Bruce's death, I didn't really know any widows in our town. The Lord has always had me with younger people which I enjoy thoroughly, but when a season of widowhood suddenly overtakes you, it can feel lonely. I couldn't imagine what Jesus would do about that! As it turned out, a wonderful close friend unexpectedly went through some very horrific circumstances with her husband that put her in a season of aloneness and grief as well. She, on her own journey of mourning, has been a wonderful gift to me and someone to walk with into a new season. We were able to do things together that you would normally do with a spouse; things like taking a vacation that would have otherwise been taken with family. None of it lessens the pain. Yet especially in the beginning, there was a fellowship of suffering that brought comfort in the midst of the loss.

CHAPTER 5

Because I process feelings best with God through writing, below is a journal entry from my writings to God as I allowed myself to work through the particular wave of grief that hit me after six months. It's very personal and might make you uncomfortable if you are not yet used to facing honest, human emotions. In Isaiah 53:3, Jesus is described as: *"A man of sorrows and acquainted with grief."* He understands our sorrow and if we will go there with him, we will not be alone, and can experience a certain kind of fellowship in the midst of our suffering. We also then have the hope that even though we will grieve, we will not *"grieve like the rest of men, who have no hope"* (Thessalonians 4:13b). We discover there is a way through to the other side of our sorrow as he walks with us in our mourning.

Jesus' promise to us: *"Blessed are those who mourn for they will be comforted"* (Matthew 5:4).

My Letter

Written to God from a deep place of grief 6 months after my husband's death:

"My Father, please direct my paths...I feel confused as to my life. Is this a part of the journey of grief? I have never been this way before and I feel restless and undone. Empty and alone. Where are you Lord? I need you so much. I feel like I am no longer on the edge of an undiscovered country as I did in the beginning of my grief, but instead now on a journey without a map, where no one has given me the directions to navigate. I feel very alone on that journey, very lost and undone. I am unable to fill the empty places with anything or anyone and feel adrift and alone without clarity and purpose – wandering in circles, very lost. I feel like a little dog wandering in circles, looking for a place to pee. Trying this and trying that, but no place satisfies the emptiness in my soul. The busyness doesn't fill it and the quietness doesn't...nothing satisfies the ache. All is

temporary, momentary. I have lots going on in my life, and it brings momentary satisfaction, but nothing lasts, remains. I am unable to take that pleasure home with me...it evaporates as soon as things end. Immediately I am thrust back into the aloneness. You are the good Shepherd who looks after and finds the lost sheep. I feel like the little lamb that is stuck in the briars – so please find me. I am wandering and trapped at the same time – it's not either one, but both and that just adds to my unsettledness and confusion. Pick me up and hold me close to your heart, Jesus. I need your comfort and strength in my weakness. I need to taste and see that you are enough in this alone season.

I need you so much. I feel lost at sea! Adrift in a big ocean, alone and yes, frightened. Even the deadly calm frightens me. That calm of the nothingness almost more so. Please come to me, come walking on the water, Jesus. I know I need to enter that deadly calm of no vision, yet the fog surrounds me, engulfs me and smothers me. I am not seeing or hearing...alone and now not even connecting deeply or intimately with you in this dark season. For so long now, I have enjoyed experiencing your intimacy, Jesus, and now I am feeling detached, separated. My experience has been Christ inside me, closer than breath and now I feel abandoned. I know you are there, waiting...for what? Me? To do what or come to what? I feel purposeless, journeyless, undone by the nothingness... What memories does all that connect to? Please show me if I need healing from the past or if this is just a new part of the grief. I don't know. I feel like I am drifting alone on that big ocean, undone by the emptiness and purposelessness.

Yet, purpose cannot be the goal. Abiding and resting, unity with you has to be the goal, otherwise I am using purpose to cover the empty places within and as a hiding place of false safety. It might work for a moment, but when new difficult circumstances come, I will be left adrift again. No, I must meet you here in this drifting lost little boat for you are my only anchor. The anchor of my soul. Otherwise my life will get trapped in people, things, work, or circumstances, and not in you. I must find my life in you again. Not just the life I found in you before my grief, but my life as it is now in the emptiness. You must become the fullness in my aching soul.

You are my way. Why am I not trusting you now to come to that place of resting and peace like I could in the beginning of my grief and loss? Why can I not just settle down now and rest in your provision? Why can I not find you here? Is this just a part of my walking through the valley of the shadow of death? Has the death of my loved one put a shadow of grief over my life that I must walk through to get to the other side of this mountain in order to discover a new way of life that comes out of union, abiding in you?

Your victory is that out of death comes resurrection life. I know that my new life is lived through your life released In me and is the hope of even my pain bringing you glory. I have experienced coming into that reality in past seasons, but is this a new season in which I must meet you as the resurrection and the life? Come, Lord Jesus, come. Come, Holy Spirit, my Comforter, come. Help me to release my hold on the old and courageously walk forward with you into my unknown future. You are my future and my hope."

After honestly pouring out my heart to Him and openly releasing my emotions, I could feel myself finally re-entering the place of peace and rest. The heaviness of heart lifted, clarity in my thinking and my soul came once again, and I experienced a return of his peace and joy within me. It became well with my soul once again.

I invite you to see if there are losses you have been grieving without your awareness. Those losses could go back many years; like the loss of a childhood because of having to grow up too fast, the death of a parent, sibling, or special person in your early years, the loss of a marriage, the loss of your health, the loss of the way you thought your life should have gone. The loss might include a marriage. You may have entered with high hopes that were dashed, and you grew angry and cold over the years, even though you are still in it. Perhaps it is a career or job that didn't ever fit you that you have continued to endure. Maybe you had a different picture for your life and future and – you had hoped... *"Hope deferred makes the heart sick..."* (Proverbs 13:12)

You might even be experiencing some of the symptoms, but without the understanding of where those symptoms have come from. If we are willing to enter our grief and walk through the process, we will come out the other side with a new acceptance and peace. Grief is a season to walk through and not just a one-time experience. However there is a vast difference between holding your grief inside and mourning the loss in order to release it.

It breaks my heart to see those who immediately jump into another relationship immediately after the loss of a marriage through divorce or death. They are then often moving into the new from a place of need. Need-based relationships are not healthy ones. Love gives, not takes, so when we can give love freely from our hearts, love is able to come back to us. However when we take or try to pull from another, we are using that person to fulfill our own needs and cover up that empty place within our own hearts. That's self-serving and the *using* of another.

Remember that Jesus said, *"Blessed are those that mourn for they will be comforted."* (Matthew 5:4) We can grieve for years with the sorrow that leads us in circles or even to self-pity and victimhood, but often our mourning has never been emotionally worked through and released. According to Scripture, there are two sorrows – one that brings "life" and one "death"; the sorrow that causes "death" must be worked through if we are going to be able to release our true sorrow and move toward "life" again. The sorrow of "death" can manifest as blame, self-pity, or depression. It can keep us trapped in anger and pain!

If we try to quickly cover over our loss with busyness or fill ourselves immediately with another relationship, the natural process can be short circuited. It's not uncommon for me to hear this statement from someone I've counseled. When I first meet with them and suggest they may have many unshed tears still buried from the past, their reply is usually, "I'm afraid if I ever start crying, I will never be able to stop". Why? They still have tears that have been buried deeply from various losses, but those tears have never been allowed to be released.

They never mourned their losses so as to come through to a new place of acceptance and peace. They live trapped in the unshed grief. It's never too late to mourn the losses of the past. As a tool, I often instruct the people who are stuck in the losses they have experienced throughout their lives to make a list of them. By doing that, they are owning their losses so they can finally be faced and released. When you face and own your grief, allowing yourself to sorrow, you get back a part of your heart that has been lost. As you listen to the words that identify the pain and connect with them, you begin the healthy process toward release and the beginning of new life and joy that comes through the sorrow.

I remember well the day, almost a year after Bruce's death, when I walked in the door, and instead of feeling alone and sad, I began to feel joy bubbles coming up from deep within my heart. My immediate thought was, "I enjoy being alone!" That new joy was only possible though, by allowing myself to be present in my grief throughout the previous months. As that new revelation of joy came, I began to realize, as Jesus did in John 16:32, that yes I was alone, but not really alone because my Father was with me.

"But a time is coming, and has come, when you will be scattered, each to his own home. You will leave me all alone. Yet I am not alone, for my Father is with me." (John 16:32)

"...Weeping may remain for a night, but rejoicing comes in the morning." (Psalm 30:5b.)

"You turned my wailing into dancing; you removed my sackcloth and clothed me with joy." (Psalm 30:11)

CHAPTER 6
Handling Our Messy Emotions and Bringing Them Under God's Control

I'm sure you've noticed that our emotions sometimes seem to have a mind of their own causing us to feel confused or tormented. Perhaps we even find our emotions shocking us at times by tumbling out unpredictably and unexpectedly. Like when you hear the tone of your voice rise and you recognize you are becoming overly defensive in a normal conversation! That can often be a sign we have simply buried certain feelings throughout the years and when triggered, they unfortunately leak out! However, far too often they can also be displaced. In that case, we are putting them on something or someone else inappropriately, and out of proportion to what is called for in the particular situation.

When we have learned, often in childhood, not to listen to our emotions, they are still there even though we no longer feel them. I have an example of displaced emotions in my last book that is sort of humorous, but also very sad. Because early on I learned not to feel, without my awareness, I was placing my buried emotions on the dog! Whenever I would leave the house for an extended period, I would fear the dog was feeling abandoned, lonely, afraid, rejected. I would experience torment. Of course those were not the dog's feelings, they were mine!

CHAPTER 6

To give another example, let's say you are feeling overly stressed at work. Or perhaps frustrated with your children, or in some other relationship. Things might be going on in your life that you have no control over and you are feeling angry, powerless, or helpless. You come home and something is out of place or someone says or does (or doesn't do) something that at another time, you would simply ignore or just speak to them kindly about, but instead you blow up! That is displaced anger. You feel out of control in a big thing that you can't do anything about, so you take it out on the next small thing or person that comes along. For example, let's say your boss was unhappy with you about something or you had an argument with your spouse. Then without even being aware, it becomes easy to pick on the children for some small offense – something you might have handled differently another time. Road rage is a good example of that! But that can simply reveal a buried anger at unfairness of any kind.

Our emotions are the voice of our hearts so if we have gotten into the habit of shutting them out, we can become unaware of the feelings we are experiencing on any deep level of the heart. We might think we know what we are feeling in our minds, but unconsciously we have created a separation between our heads and hearts so a very different set of emotions are brewing within. This could have happened because emotions were not considered acceptable in our particular family growing up or we might have been shamed for them and told things like, *"Get over it!"*, *"Don't cry!"* Sometimes our emotions simply felt too confusing or painful and we didn't know how to handle them because few of us were taught how to process them in a healthy way.

The unfortunate reality is that if our parents never accepted their own feelings, they had nothing to give to us in that regard. You can only give what you have. To add to that disappointment is the truth that we were created for relationships with our hearts engaged, but when our emotions get shut down we can no longer live our lives from there. The result is that our relationships begin to become superficial and we might begin to *pull* on others to fill us. I always knew when my husband was shutting down his heart because his conversation would then become about the weather! I used to joke about it. As we close off our hearts, our passions deaden and we often find ourselves beginning to live with a vague sense of dissatisfaction or emptiness that can leave us feeling disconnected and lonely. When that happens, it's not unusual for us to try to wrongly *"pull"* on others to fill the emptiness. On top of that, sometimes our suppressed passions will begin to come out sideways and we find ourselves going after anything that seems to satisfy the emptiness. That causes us to further distance from our hearts and deaden our real desires.

This happens far too frequently in marriages. Let's say the normal hurts and disagreements of life are never fully faced and grieved. Without owning them, they cannot be released to the place of heart forgiveness so they just quietly build one on top of another deep inside. Before long there are dividing walls of hostility and resentment being erected within. Forgiveness never just overlooks the offense by simply excusing the other, or by putting the hurt under the carpet. It instead requires us to look squarely at the pain it caused us, yet then release it to God, allowing him to meet us in that hurt with his healing love. As we face our emotions in that way, we are often then able to talk about it without an emotional over-reaction or displacing our anger. Jesus was wounded in every way such as we have been – same emotions, just different circumstances, so he can connect with our hearts in our own suffering. The Bible refers to that as a fellowship of suffering. In that fellowship, we are no longer left alone in our pain.

CHAPTER 6

Peace At Any Cost Is Not Peace

Too often we either try to keep the hurt and anger buried under the carpet of self-control or settle for a peace that pacifies and involves the selling of our souls to keep another happy. We don't want to rock our already fragile boat. In Matthew 10:34-39, we find Jesus saying that he didn't come to bring peace but a sword – sometimes that sword cuts open and reveals that which the false peace would try to cover. In marriage this plays out frequently. In order to get a momentary respite, that is not really true peace at all, the temptation is to keep things under the carpet for the illusion of peace. Sadly, that tactic simply places another brick of cold resentment over our hearts. We are, unfortunately, just burying our anger or hurt feelings. As the years go on, we have built a fortress without realizing it, until sadly, the once felt passion has been replaced with cold-hearted contempt. The contempt is actually just our buried anger leaking out. Contempt by definition is disdain, lack of respect, and concealed anger that can come out in a hurtful attitude or tone, even in sarcastic joking. The question that may be formed, although deeply hidden in the heart and usually not articulated is, *"Why did I ever marry this person?" "What was I thinking?"*

"Love must be sincere. Hate what is evil, cling to what is good." (Romans 12:9)

When we finally face the reality of how the enemy of our souls, the destroyer, has used incident after incident to destroy what was once our most precious relationship, the scripture from Ephesians 4:26 about not allowing the sun to go down on your anger begins to make sense. It doesn't say not to be angry – anger is a human emotion that is needed, but we have to discover why we are really angry and not just blame the other. Maturity allows us to separate the person's true heart from the survival system they are currently exhibiting and not just attack the other, but deal with the unhealthy system itself.

We can then begin to recognize the disappointed desires that are fueling our anger and face our sadness. If honest, both partners usually have disappointments that need to be talked through. We identify and share the disappointed desires hiding under the anger so that each can take their own responsibility for intentionally, or even unintentionally, hurting the other by something they have done or neglected to do. When we hurt someone we love even without meaning to, we are meant to feel sorrow, not defensiveness. Unhealed false shame can cause us to feel powerless, then get angry from feeling exposed, instead of accepting that in our humanity, we have failed or hurt another. Feeling our sorrow over having hurt the one we love, allows us to feel legitimate shame, and then ask for forgiveness from the heart.

Because we all have a deep longing or desire to be known, seen, and heard, when we are not being heard, we feel disregarded. Almost like we don't matter and then we feel we must defend ourselves. It has been my experience that if you boil down most hurts and disagreements between couples, you will find that underneath it all, one or even both, do not feel really known, valued, heard, or seen by the other. We get so busy defending the fact we are *right* in our disagreements that we forget life is not meant to be about being *right*, but it is meant instead to be *life-giving*. Being right comes from the wrong tree, the Tree of the Knowledge of Good and Evil. When we really listen to someone and hear their heart, even when we don't agree, we give them value and respect. That is the Tree of Life! Then when we share how we are feeling, they are more prone to listen even if in the end you have to agree to disagree. It's not about *right and wrong* but about *life and death!* When we really hear the hurt a seemingly insignificant act (to us) caused another, we are meant to have empathy. Then we can connect with an open heart, asking for

CHAPTER 6

forgiveness for causing the pain even though it might just have been thoughtless or unintentional.

Healthy relationships are built on honor and respect so, if we don't really listen to the hurt of another, we are not really respecting their heart. Remember, our feelings, good, bad, or ugly are expressing what is currently happening on the heart level and are not usually logical, but emotional. That's why it is so helpful to process them alone with God emotionally before trying to talk to the other about them. I find it helpful to write a letter to that person first – one they will never see! Once the feelings have been processed, it is much easier to talk rationally and with empathy instead of anger.

When someone would do something that was irresponsible, hurtful, or neglectful, my husband who was very responsible, would usually try to understand logically why they would act so irresponsibly or make such an unfortunate choice. Knowledge can often be a form of control. Our needing to know why or try to understand their reasoning can often be an act of our own need to feel in control. When people are acting out of past unhealed issues in their lives, they will not act in a logical way so it will not make any sense if you try to figure it out. When people are acting out emotionally, any logic usually goes out the window!

I had a long-standing habit of burying my anger instead of acknowledging it. How many times, years ago, did I say, "I'm not angry", when unknown to me at the time, I was full of buried rage. That anger had been building inside of me throughout the years of marriage. In those days, I felt powerless, voiceless, and controlled, so I became controlling. On the outside I was nice, even though it was still laced with hidden contempt until... the explosions were far between, but they came when the straw finally broke the camel's back. Each time I had buried my anger prior to the explosion had simply added to my building resentment and became another brick that separated us on a deep level of the heart.

That unacknowledged anger within is like a poison in our soul. It eventually affects our bodies as well, in various ways, like headaches or other aches and pains, arthritis, skin conditions, intestinal issues, the list goes on and on. It can also come out sideways as a tone in the voice, impatience, disguised put-downs, a superior attitude, or in shaming the other. In the heart there often lurks a contemptuous attitude and buried disdain.

Anger is a covering emotion like the lid on a box. Take the lid off and what do you find in the box? There may be disappointments of all kinds, fears, smashed hopes and dreams, feelings of helplessness or of being out of control. Maybe at the same time we feel controlled by the other, trapped, or perhaps unseen or heard, not valued or encouraged. Holding onto our anger helps us to feel so much more powerful and in control. Those struggling emotions we've tucked away in our box make us feel powerless, helpless, disappointed, sad, trapped and unable to fix anything. However if we will acknowledge the feelings that have been pushed away, share them with God, and then begin to learn to communicate from a place of sorrow instead of anger, both partners have an opportunity to grow together and really get to know each other on the heart level. It is messy for sure because emotions are a mess, but they also reveal the status of our hearts. Jesus longs to make beauty out of ashes as Isaiah 61 reminds us.

Why do we want so badly to control a situation or a person? Control usually stems from fear so when we've experienced the uncertainties of living with a parent's addiction or abuse of any kind, it can become a way of life. Fear, uncertainty, insecurity and feelings of powerlessness are usually the underlying emotions. Especially if we have pushed away any experience of feeling out of control, helpless, rejected, abandoned, used, abused or trapped as a child, we can carry a buried fear of those particular emotions ever again surfacing. We might have been hurt by one parent who was abusive while the other sat idly by, never protecting us, so we learned to control our own world. Control became our only survival at the time, and by trying to control our world, we got the illusion of safety, security. When we were children, we thought like children, but now as adults we need to release those childish ways, as the scripture reminds us, because they are sabotaging our relationships.

When we are willing to face ourselves and the hurts still buried within our hearts, we begin to connect with our true selves. We actually begin to become ourselves – our real selves – as we allow Jesus to come into those hurts. As a man on this earth, Jesus suffered in every way such as we do, so he could become a faithful high priest for us. As we face our pain, he understands, and Jesus who knew the agony firsthand, is able to come along side us – not with just sympathy, but with true empathy. Sympathy looks down on, feels sorry for, but empathy comes alongside and connects on a heart level. We develop an intimacy with Jesus as we fellowship with him in our suffering. That allows him to weep with us as a *"Man of Sorrows acquainted with suffering"*. And by his stripes (his pain) we are healed as we allow him to share with us in our own suffering and sorrows. (Isaiah 53)

Just a study in the gospels of the last week of Jesus' life reveals the emotional horror that Jesus experienced. He was rejected, despised, betrayed, disowned, mocked, laughed at, misunderstood, falsely accused, abused, and shamed. Life was not fair for Jesus, yet he was perfect, he did no wrong. Jesus was left alone with deep disappointment after requesting his disciples just sit with him for one hour, but they didn't ever really hear him. They promptly fell asleep, neglecting his longing for companionship as he went through the deepest wrestling of his life. Throughout that experience of having to surrender to his Father's will and walk through the horror that lay ahead, Jesus was so overcome with anguish that he sweat blood out of his pores while his friends continued to sleep on oblivious to his agony. Jesus longed for their fellowship in his suffering, but they were not there for him in the worst moments of his life. That has also been the experience for many of us – feeling left all alone and misunderstood when we needed those we loved the most, but they were sadly absent. Jesus not only felt abandoned by his friends, but even by his God and Father in those horrific moments on the cross. He understands! Because of that, we now have one guaranteed relationship in which we will never again be rejected or abandoned no matter whatever else happens to us in this life. Because he has experienced all those emotions and more, and he desires to fellowship with us in our sufferings, we will never be left all alone again.

At the end of John 16:32, we find Jesus sorrowfully sharing these words with his disciples. They were some of the last words he spoke to them before his death as Jesus stood facing the horror that was to come. He said, *"You will leave me all alone. Yet I am not alone, for my Father is with me."* As we are willing to work through our own disappointed desires and sorrows, those same words begin to ring true to us emotionally in ways we could only understand in an intellectual way before.

Emotions are part of our humanity. They are to be embraced simply because they are ours, not necessarily to be lived out of, but to be owned, accepted. We all have good, bad, and ugly in us and we will continue to have as long as we live with this flesh. Flesh is flesh and it can be very ugly at times, even in Christians. By facing that reality, we are actually moving toward healing and the release of the bad and the ugly. However, if we push the emotions down or ignore them, we can develop a false life that causes us to hide our true selves and live behind a mask. We can't clean up the flesh by covering it over – flesh is flesh, but we can begin to live an authentic life from the heart as we join with the Spirit; honestly facing ourselves and then participating in his

CHAPTER 6

sanctifying, purifying, healing work in the deepest, ugliest recesses of our hearts.

One of the main things God seems to use to complete this process within us happens to be our circumstances. Going through difficult circumstances in any important area of life has a way of bringing to the surface those things we have tried to push away. Emotions such as fear of the outcome of something that is important to us can cause our insecurities to rise up along with the accompanying anxiety. It's not unusual then to find yourself distracted and out of sorts. We might even experience anger at God, or perhaps even quiet terror as we look ahead at what might happen that we can't control. At that point, it may be that our formerly hidden, unspoken question begins to surface within us, *"Where are you, God?"* That question is often followed by a silent, often hidden, demand of the heart, *"I need you to fix this now!"*

Too often we have a buried belief that these things are not supposed to be happening to us, and the truth is, in a perfect world they wouldn't. That lie can come out of a very limited view of God and his ways, as well as a lack of understanding of the broken world we currently live in. One day at Jesus' return there will be justice, but not here. Isaiah tells us that God's ways are higher than ours so we can't bring him down to our way of thinking, we can't even pray him down! We must go to him to learn his ways, and quite honestly, his ways can sometimes feel pretty scary! For those of us who wanted to hold our own world together, it can feel very frightening at first because we are no longer under our own control. However, there is great freedom in releasing our lives to the only one who truly holds all things together!

When we are faced with surrender, we find out how little we really trust God on a deep heart level. Our heads trust, yes, but where the rubber meets the road, we are terrified! So then the question becomes, *"God, are you really good?"* That is a question too few of us wrestle with on any deep level of the heart, but a necessary question to struggle with emotionally. Logic reveals that we will not deeply trust and rest in someone we are afraid of or don't trust. When we try to control it's because we don't really trust God. Does he really work all things together for our good or not?

Look at 1 John 4:18,19 paraphrased in the L.B. *"We need have no fear of someone who loves us perfectly; his perfect love for us eliminates all dread of what he might do to us. If we are afraid, it is for fear of what he might do to us and shows that we are not fully convinced that he really loves us."* So you see, our love for him comes as a result of our accepting and being able to trust and rest in *his* deep love for us first. Then our love for others comes from beginning to love and accept ourselves as he loves and cares for us. As we love ourselves as he does, we begin to love and care for others from the right starting place – the experience of his love in our lives even when we don't deserve it! As we receive God's undeserved grace, we are able to give grace to others and allow him to be their judge instead of us.

We often think we are trusting God when we believe with our heads, but Jesus tells us it's with the *heart* man believes. That's why it often takes adverse circumstances to reveal to us what we are really fearing and believing deep within. When we are unable to rest in his good purposes for us, we usually get angry and afraid. Too often then, we either shut down in depression or try to control something, anything – other people, ourselves, our circumstances, or even God himself! Wrestling with these questions and facing any anger we might be silently harboring toward God is of upmost importance if we are to go on in genuine faith. Honesty and openness with God and ourselves is necessary if we are to come to a peace that remains. God knows our hearts far more deeply than we know ourselves so he is never surprised or shocked at our anger. Most Christians are afraid to admit the true anger they have with God, and so instead, shut it down, pretending they're not angry. That creates a religiosity and a distant, dishonest relationship with God, not the intimate one, our hearts and his, really desire.

Psalm 103:14 reminds us, *"He knows how we are formed, he remembers that we are dust"*. He remembers that we are made from the clay of the ground as Genesis 2 reveals, and that our true life only comes from God's Spirit within us. Even as Christians we all have tracts of our personality that have been covered over, often through shame and the hurts of the past, and have been buried deeply in denial. Sadly, those parts have not yet been faced and submitted to the Spirit's control because we can only surrender that which we know. As a result, we are unable to live in *that area* from the life of God's Spirit, but instead we live from our buried fears. I often joke that my gift of evangelism is to bring Jesus to the hidden places in the hearts of God's people that have never yet been evangelized!

If we are to fulfill our personal stories in the way God originally intended, bear fruit with our lives that will last for eternity, and become the people he was acquainted with even before we were born, we need to become wholly submitted to him and his purposes for us. Those are the purposes that will free us to live creatively from the center of our beings, and will satisfy us most deeply because they fit us! To do that though, we must be willing to take the sometimes hard, often painful, yet deeply satisfying journey of discovering our true selves. I met with someone today who told me she was now finally on a wonderful, at times painful, journey that was for the first time bringing her a taste of real life in spite of its difficulty. She was beginning to feel more alive than she ever had, and felt she was moving toward really living the life she was created to live.

When I begin meeting with someone, they come to me more often than not, if not hating, at least strongly disliking parts of themselves. They might like their gifts or strengths, but have rejected their hearts. As they become willing to walk further down the journey of healing, at some point I begin to see their countenance change. It's at that point I will ask the question, "Do you like being you?" Formerly their answer had been, "I hate being me!", but now their response is mostly an enthusiastic, "I love being me, I wouldn't want to be anyone else!" Lori, who I met with just this past week shared she was discovering exciting parts of herself she never knew existed. She wasn't yet fully loving herself, but was beginning to know and enjoy who she was discovering. It's always amazing to me how little of ourselves we have really known until beginning the journey of discovery!

Our Longings and Desires

If we are to become who we really are, we must sort through any illegitimate shame we are carrying and rediscover our longings and our deepest desires. They are good, even though often disappointed. Our longings are at the deepest part of our being and can only fully be filled by God himself for this is still a very broken world. The lies and demands that have overtaken us must be recognized and released so they can be replaced by the truth of God's word. You cannot put truth on top of a lie and expect it to remain – the lie must first be faced and released, with all its accompanying pain, so a new foundation of truth can be built in our innermost being. Psalm 51:6 reminds us that God desires truth in our inner parts, not just in our minds. Our foundations, and how they have been built upon, are important to God. If the foundation is faulty, the whole building will be affected. Recently, as I was praying about a situation close to my heart, God revealed the reason for this couple's present trouble was that the marriage had been originally been built on fear and anger. That fear and anger didn't begin in the marriage, it only played out there for it began in childhood for each of them.

CHAPTER 6

The shame that comes in through any form of abuse will affect us in every way, each and every day of our lives, even when we are not aware of it. I can't begin to tell you how many lives I have seen, still imprisoned through unhealed abuse, even though they have had much emotional healing and deliverance in other areas. Abuse sabotages our lives and holds us captive. Unhealed past abuse colors our choices and can cause us to make bad decisions. It affects the way we treat ourselves and how we try to *pull* from others – it drives the systems we use to survive, often at another's expense. It can be the driving force behind our shame, often causing pride, and how we will try to prove ourselves to others so we can feel valuable. It can cause us to wear a mask and hide our true hearts in shame and unworthiness. I personally have never seen a person get full victory until their former abuse has been faced, along with the accompanying shame that was never theirs to begin with, released.

The truth that replaces our personal false-identity lie is the Spirit of Christ himself who longs to take up residence in the deepest part of our broken heart where the shame lie has been living. That wondrous blessing can happen as we finally become willing to face our lies, release them, and meet Jesus there with his healing touch. Jesus suffered similar feelings of abuse, rejection, abandonment, and shame so he could connect with us there. By his wounds, we can be healed. (Isaiah 53) As we do that, an exchange is made in the deep recesses of our hearts – his acceptance for our shame. We can't serve two masters at the depth of our being, it will be either the shame that abusively drives us through the dark lies of the enemy or Jesus who gently leads us into all truth, light, acceptance, value, and love.

The shame lies or false beliefs we have gotten trapped in have often taken up residence in our lives through others' anger, betrayals, rejections, and the shame we have experienced through the hands of another. Instrumental people in our lives have taught us how to see and treat ourselves by the way they treated us. I recently saw a powerful TV program where a mother acknowledged to her emotionally damaged son that she made him a container for her own rage! She was so angry within her own life, she spewed it out on her son in rage. That rage gave him a false identity based on the message that he was bad and worthless. He became just a scapegoat.

How can we heal from things like that? When we can begin to recognize that is not who we really are, and refuse to continue to self-reject, we can begin to meet our true selves perhaps for the first time! As we begin to allow God's Spirit to surface the lies, we are then able to get out of agreement with the enemy of our souls against ourselves. Unfortunately, we have learned how to treat ourselves by the way others have treated us throughout our lives. Finally, as we face the pain and accept God's loving truth, the door is opened for us to align ourselves with Jesus. He is the author and finisher of our faith, who is the way, the truth, and our very life, the one who called us from before we were ever born. Sadly though, until embarking on a healing journey, many of us have learned to listen instead to the accuser of the brethren (Satan, the enemy) who has been accusing us day and night, feeding the thoughts and lies that were already lodged within.

Taking Back Our Story

We must take our lives back from where we have given them over to people or things to find whatever morsels of life we could eek out to fill the hole in our hearts. Only God and his love and acceptance of us can fill that hole. As we begin to recognize that and take our lives back bit by bit, Jesus invites us to release to him each new part we have discovered. Until getting our lives back, we don't fully have our hearts to give him because almost everyone and everything else has a piece of us. Far too often, we don't even realize it because we have

CHAPTER 6

locked our wounded emotions away, even from ourselves. We can only truly surrender to him that which we know and have accepted. Whatever is still buried within is not yet ours to release to God.

It is like having locked closets in our home that have been filled with trash. We can clean the rest of the house, but until those closets are unlocked and opened, we cannot sort out what is trash. Until I personally sorted through the "locked closets" within me, the actual closets in my home were always in disarray! I have watched many who, as they began to finally sort through and release the buried clutter in their lives, begin to have the desire and energy to bring order to the messes in their homes.

As we begin the process of rediscovering those parts of us that have been lost, and as we are willing to release them to him, our journey becomes an amazing ongoing process of wonder, enjoyment, and getting to know the person God has always k own. The one he has always loved. That is the one Jesus wept over, longed for, and waited to heal. He has been quietly knocking on the door of our each of our hearts, calling to us to trust him enough to invite him into those areas of hurt and pain. He desires to fellowship with us in our suffering and heal our wounded hearts. He then calls us go with him in the wonderfully unique way we were designed so we can co-labor with him in a much larger story than we ever imagined.

Jesus can't do it for us, but he invites us to join with him in discovering that little one locked within who has been lost for a very long time, struggling through, just trying to survive. The self-rejection didn't begin in the adult self, but usually goes all the way back into early childhood, if not beginning even in the womb or at birth. We can be born into an atmosphere of rejection, shame, and abandonment – I know I was. Since we learn from others how to treat ourselves, if we felt rejected or shamed by significant others, we learned to treat ourselves in the same manner.

As a result, the real person within us, has gotten lost. Jesus came to seek that which was lost. We see him in Scripture depicted as the good Shepherd who goes after that one little lamb who has been stuck in the thicket afraid and alone. The one he desires to rescue is who Psalm 139 describes as fearfully and wonderfully made – that's you! God made that declaration while you were still in the womb of your mother before any of the robbery of a broken world occurred. Jesus longs to reveal to us how our chapters, even the painful parts, fit into the story he has been telling throughout history. Our lives are meant to release the unique treasures God has placed within us into a hurting world. However for many of us, those treasures have remained dormant and undiscovered, still locked within. I never saw the treasures God had placed within me and as long as I compared myself with others, I felt worthless. It takes a willingness for us to join him on the search for our true selves if we are ever to discover our own buried treasures. God desires to restore the days ordained for us that have been robbed through simply living in a fallen world – those are the days Jesus came to redeem. (Psalm 139:13-16) Our lives matter in a far larger way than we could ever have imagined!

The question he asks each of us to answer not from just our heads, but in our hearts, is – are we willing to trust him enough to take a journey with him back through our original story to find that little one within who is still stuck, lost, and derailed from their story? That story was written for them from before the foundation of the world. I'm sure I haven't yet gotten my whole story back, but I have gotten enough of it to know that I am fully enjoying the person I am becoming and the story that is now unfolding before me! I am doing far more than I ever thought possible, not as a performance, but with ease, simply allowing those rivers of living water to be released from my innermost being. It amazingly is effortless!

Where others go and who they touch is his business, not mine. My part is to work with God's Spirit to allow that living water to flow freely in the way he designed me.

Jesus' mission was and still is to heal the broken hearted and bring beauty out of ashes, Isaiah 61 reminds us. He is the only one who can take the mess of our lives and find the buried treasure, the jewels that have been hidden deeply in the ashes of our lives. However that is always a co-labor so we must be willing to join with him on the treasure hunt! We often fall into a ditch on either side of the road – either we pray and pray for him to fix us, or get into another self-help program. It is only when we join with him on our own behalf that we find true change begins. Most of us have spent far too many years either trying to prove ourselves to people through performing or in self-condemnation. It is time to direct our anger toward the true enemy who has tried to rob us. We do that by fighting *for our lives* instead of self-sabotaging against ourselves or others in blame.

"The thief comes only to steal and kill and destroy; I have come that they may have life to the full", Jesus declares. (John 10:10) Our cooperation with God in deep inner healing, is meant to bring us to a new place of surrender and trust in God and his wondrous purposes for our lives. But it requires the discovery of *his* purposes for us, in *his* way, not ours. Allowing the amazing healing of our own brokenheartedness that came in through the rejections, betrayals, and shaming abandonments we experienced, enables us to release the grip we have had on our own lives and the false pictures we have painted for ourselves. The healing of our wounded hearts allows us to place ourselves more and more into his safe, loving hands. As we do, our ability to trust and risk begins to grow.

The purpose of getting our lives back is so we can freely and joyfully release them back to God for his purposes. That process involves laying down our own willfulness and allowing him to implant his good will and purposes for us into our hearts. *"For it is God who works in you to will and to act according to his good purpose."* (Philippians 2:13) We can then begin to live a shared adventure for his glory and purpose, and not just for our own survival and agenda. We will die to self only to discover that it's not death at all, but actually resurrection life, and we will find an amazing walk with him that travels on *his* highway not ours, joyfully filling our soul. We will become able to allow God to break our hearts with the things that break his.

Through the eyes of our hearts being opened, we can begin to see others in a way that loves the person's true heart while at the same time, still hates the evil systems they might be using. *"Hate what is evil, love what is good",* the Bible reminds us. We are meant to hate what God hates – never the person, but always the evil, the robbery, the survival systems that are used whether they be control, anger, abuse, or any other thing of that nature. Those systems are meant to be hated, even in ourselves. Yet at the same time, the person's true heart is to be loved, sought after, and fought for. Sometimes that can only be done in prayer, but also with a refusal to get trapped in the games they are still playing. It takes two to play a game – if one quits, the game is over! *"Love must be sincere. Hate what is evil; cling to what is good."* (Romans 12:9) (Isaiah 61:8 & Amos 5:14,15)

With joy we begin to get our story back and see the beautiful significance he has given to our own very personal lives. At last we begin to recognize that it is truly his desire to redeem the painful parts of our lives and weave them into the story our lives are now telling. We begin to enjoy being the person he has created and become willing to allow him to fit our story into his storyline. Our story is meant to fit very wonderfully and uniquely into HIS-STORY. That is the story he is re-writing as the Author of all things. He is the author and the finisher of our story. But we are to fit into his plans, not the other way around! As we allow that, our lives begin

CHAPTER 6

to bring him ever increasing glory. *"Christ in us the hope of glory."* (Col. 1:27) In the Scripture, over and over shame is seen as the opposite of glory. As any legitimate shame we might still be carrying from the past is faced, it is forgiven through Jesus' sacrifice on the cross. Then any false shame we've carried illegitimately for another can be released to the one to whom it really belongs, and then Jesus' glory is able to begin to take its place. (Psalm 4:2)

If you have children, you might recognize the various gifts and treasures within them, but if they were to continue to live their lives by hiding and sabotaging those treasures you would feel sad. However, when your children finally discover who they really are and start to release those gifts and treasures, you would feel great joy. Then as you thought of your children, you would feel proud of them for becoming their true selves. That's the joy our heavenly Father experiences over his kids as they finally begin to become who he originally created them to be! His face shines on us with the words, *"This is my son, or my daughter who makes my heart glad for their very being brings me glory"*.

CHAPTER 7
Uncovering Our Own Hearts and Discovering the Essence of Who We Really Are

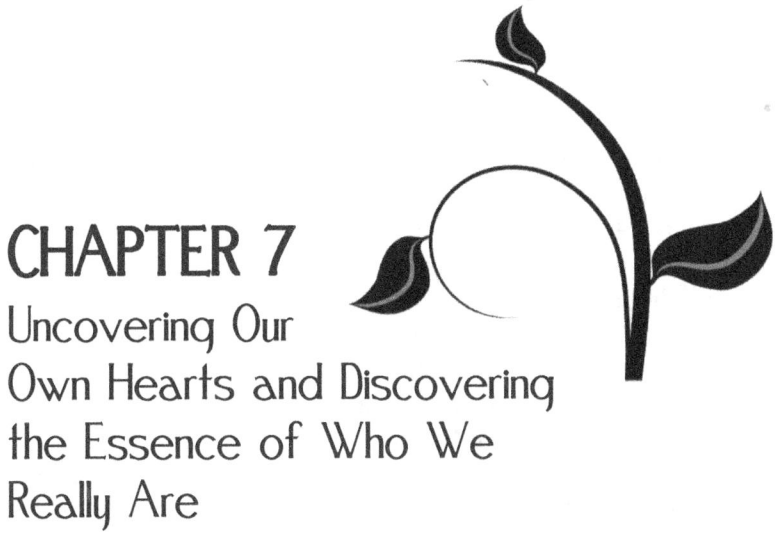

Our hearts are central – that is a truth in the spiritual and emotional parts of our lives as well as in our physical bodies. In the physical if our hearts shut down we die. The same can be true in the spiritual and emotional realms except that far too often we are not even aware we have died. When we close down due to the hurts and pain we've experienced in our hearts, we can begin to live from outside of ourselves mostly without even realizing it. Sadly then we begin to be directed by others, or by our circumstances, and we become more humans doing than human beings because we have disconnected from the very life flow of our hearts.

As a result, we are frequently drawn to performing and trying to please others or we become controllers and just try to hold everything together. Life can too often then begin to feel like drudgery that eventually burns us out instead of being a life-giving experience. Out of our inmost being (the heart) comes real life and true connection with others, including God. When we as Christians shut down our hearts, God doesn't leave, but at that point he often feels distant or

CHAPTER 7

far off, because we are no longer connecting with him from inside ourselves on the heart level.

When our hearts shut down, our true self is buried and our connection with others can become superficial instead of from the heart. I could always tell when my husband was shutting down because as we sat together at the end of the day, the conversation would become about nothingness! What at another time would be a much more meaningful time of sharing, now felt empty. That is true of our connection with God as well, and it's then that other things and temptations begin to have more and more of an appeal. We have lost the essence of our own true selves but rarely realize it. Jesus spoke of loving God with our *whole heart, mind, soul, and strength*, but it takes a heart connection to do that. Otherwise we are going through the motions outwardly, doing all the right things perhaps, but our hearts remain lost and locked up within.

In the past, I used to lose my heart quite often and it took recognizing that lost feeling to even understand I had shut my heart down. As I became aware of what I was doing when I distanced from what my heart was telling me through my emotions (either good or bad), I made the joyful discovery that Jesus wasn't afar off at all, as I was feeling he was. He was still within me... patiently waiting. It was I who had moved away when I distanced myself from my heart. As soon as I would allow myself, with the Spirit's help, to discover what my heart was trying to speak through my feelings whether good, bad, or ugly, and simply *acknowledge* those emotions (not live from them), I was back within my own heart immediately. I began to recognize that God hadn't moved, I had!

As I reconnected with my heart, I discovered the joyous truth that the Spirit of Jesus was there awaiting my return! Once again we had intimate connection, even in the sometimes ugliness of my emotions, but now I could talk with him about my struggle and invite him to help me work it through. If there was someone I needed to forgive, Jesus the forgiver would patiently work with me there even if it took some time for me to finally arrive at the point of heart forgiveness. Too often we forgive others out of duty from our minds alone, but our hearts continue to remain shut down from that person. We might even be "nice" on the outside, but in reality, we are still closed toward them on the inside.

It's from the heart we love. It's in the heart we receive love. When are hearts are still broken, even when we hear of God's love for us, that truth is unable to find a place to remain. We are unable to stay connected to his incredible love for long. When others share good words about us, we might get even puffed up for a moment in pride, but then because of the lies within, any truth that was spoken to us seldom remains. Having our broken hearts healed and then exchanging the former lies for God's truth, opens us up to receive God's love, to actively love him back, and then begin to truly love and accept others with his love.

I share this statement from Rick Joyner: *"Loving God is the first and greatest commandment, yet this love is not just an emotion. The word used for "love" in this commandment is not a noun but a verb, an action word. You cannot command an emotion in others. Therefore, our goal must not be to sequester ourselves in a place where we can just sit and feel emotions for God, but our love for God should be the controlling factor in our lives, in all that we do."* Healing enables us to move into action, co-laboring with God, on the heart level. We begin to sense his compassion in various circumstances instead of either just our own human compassion or our judgments.

The healing of our broken hearts though can sometimes be a very painful or difficult process for us, so it's natural we want to avoid. However, it's not a process we enter alone. God wants to walk with us through it so we are no longer left alone in our past or present struggles. A very practical way of reconnecting with your heart is to write about your feelings – not your thoughts, but your emotions! That can be difficult at first because of the disconnection, but remember your feelings are the voice of your heart. Consequently, if you begin to discover what you are really feeling on the heart level, you are reconnecting. Determining to write from your feelings instead of from your thoughts can help, but at first you might not have much success. In the back of the book, you will find a partial feeling list to aid you in the process. When I first began to do that about 25 years ago, I had no clue what I was feeling so I began to ask God to show me. My writings, at that time, consisted of more questions than feelings or answers, but by persevering over time, I wonderfully reconnected with my heart.

There is another danger regarding the heart that we must be aware of if we continue to shut it down, and that is a decreasing sensitivity or the hardening of our hearts. In Ephesians 4:18,19, we see a downward spiral that begins with our heart sensitivity shutting down. As a result of that heart hardening, it tells us we will become darkened in our understanding and separated from the vibrant life of God. We will begin to lose our former sensitivity, eventually giving ourselves over to sensuality. A dictionary definition of sensuality: pertaining to the senses. In other words, we will begin to be ruled by the lust of our senses. If we choose to remain hardened, the Scripture tells us, it can spiral even further toward indulging in every kind of impurity with a continual lust for more. That is the pathway of various addictions.

"Above all else, guard your heart, for it is the wellspring of life." (Proverbs 4:23) When we begin to see the value of our own hearts, we will see how important it is to watch over them carefully so they don't get lost or hardened. We begin to see that guarding them is to be done above all else for they are the most precious part of us and the key to real living! I find that for me, it is necessary to write my letter to God each day,

sharing my feelings in order to remain connected. Otherwise it can be in as little as three days without that I begin to lose the deepest connection with my own heart.

What caused our hearts to get lost in the first place? The hurts of life, the painful situations we endured throughout our lives have caused us to shut them down and so we automatically begin to live from our heads alone and from outside of our hearts. Wounded people wound people, that's just a fact of life – Christian or not. In fact, for many of us, most of our past hurts came from either family, friends, or the church. That is why the healing of our broken hearts (not heads) is so important and was Jesus' mission. When we've been hurt, we self-protect. We put a cover over our hearts to remain safe and then as hurts accumulate, much energy is spent on remaining intact, keeping ourselves safe from feeling the past hurts. As I meet with people, I laughingly refer to it as simply taking out the trash. It is simply releasing the hurt, rejection, and unforgiveness of the past that has weighed down our hearts and caused them to remain lost and hidden under a cover of self-protection.

Far too many times, we as people become so focused on protecting ourselves that we only see others in how they relate to us. Let me tell you what I mean. I hear from so many I counsel words to this effect, "She snubbed me", or "I don't think he/she likes me very much." When I ask why they feel that way, it becomes apparent that it was really just a perception they picked up from the atmosphere surrounding their friend. At that point, they might have been correctly reading the atmosphere, but what if that friend was not feeling well or just having a bad day and at that moment was focused inward? In that case we are not seeing the other at all, but only how we are feeling. That selfishness can sometimes spring from our past rejections that have never been faced and healed. We are then putting the past on the present and making a judgment that might not be at all accurate. Our perceptions often get skewed if we view life

CHAPTER 7

starting with ourselves. From the starting place of self, we are unable to truly see the other at all, but are really just focusing on how we feel, which unconsciously can put a self-protective wall around our heart. Then we become hyper-vigilant, on guard, self-protectors instead of entrusting ourselves to God.

Becoming healthy in our relationships involves first loving, seeing, and accepting ourselves as God sees, knows, loves, and accepts us – he *sees* and *knows* all of us including the good, bad, and ugly yet still loves and accepts us. *"And the second (commandment) is like it: Love your neighbor as* (you love) *yourself."* (Matthew 22:39). The journey of learning to love others as God loves them begins, not by beating ourselves up or putting "should's" on ourselves, but by seeing and accepting God's love for us even when we are in our most ugly moment! Becoming able to see others from God's heart and perspective comes from our being able to see ourselves without pretense and still love ourselves because God does even though it's not deserved. What we truly have earned is hell, but Jesus paid the ultimate sacrifice by taking our punishment for us.

When we are willing to see all our own ugliness and yet realize that God's love for us is still fully there at that moment, though totally undeserved, amazingly opens the door to our hearts. As we do that, we can begin to see another in their ugliness or unworthiness and still accept them. It has been very helpful in my own process of accepting and learning to love myself to stop when I have just been at my worst moment and say, *"Thank you God that you love me right now just the way I am, even though I don't deserve it."* For years I felt terrible guilt over having a very judgmental, critical spirit which I tried desperately to get rid of. Accepting myself with all my flaws became the key to finally releasing it. However whenever the acceptance and love of myself begins to slip, I will then begin the downward slide of seeing others through that old critical and judgmental spirit. When I recognize that, I realize I am falling away from loving myself, and the natural result is, I become unable to continue to love others.

One of the things that prevents us from receiving God's love in the first place are the judgments we have made concerning ourselves. If we have deeply judged ourselves for years, it is our normal default to either treat ourselves as unacceptable or to falsely exalt ourselves. It is common then to use words against ourselves like unacceptable, not valuable, a failure, not measuring up, etc. Those are shaming words that condemn us when God assures us in Romans 8:1 that there is *no longer any condemnation for those who are in Christ Jesus!* In some cases, the other side of the coin of non-acceptance of self might look very different by causing a person to see themselves as being more than others and exalt themselves above. That is just the pride side coming out of the same root of a shame-based identity.

Our Imaginations Reclaimed

Our imaginations create all sorts of pictures whether good or bad. For example, if your spouse is long overdue in returning from a trip, the imagination often pictures all sorts of things like a car crash or some other tragedy. If he or she has been aloof, distant, or emotionally absent lately, you might even conjure up a picture of them having an affair. Perhaps your child is not answering his cell phone after you have called him several times and his curfew was well over an hour ago. He might be a new driver so all sorts of pictures play on your mind, especially if he is usually punctual. As a result of the twisted journey our imagination has just taken, various fearful emotions begin to build within the heart so then the pictures we create (with the enemy's willing help) influence our emotions even more. Since our emotions are the voice of the heart, our heart often begins to take a journey of fear and terror. At that point the temptation is often to begin to

CHAPTER 7

convince ourselves otherwise by using our mind to push the emotion away and lock down our heart even further. Or we immediately go to the emotion we feel most powerful in like anger that covers up the fear of our powerlessness. Then when the child finally arrives home, we lash out in anger instead of just being able to voice our concern.

We first need to acknowledge that our heart is suddenly filled with fear, but then also tell ourselves the truth that we have no proof of anything like that happening, and until we do, we choose not to entertain those pictures. We choose not to run ahead of any legitimate information we presently have. That then becomes a good time to begin to praise God that he holds all things together so no matter what might happen, he has it all in his hands already, and we don't have to take control. However if we are so emotionally distraught that we are unable to choose that option, our fear is usually coming from a past loss or situation that could go back as far as early childhood. It might even be coming from an atmosphere of fear and insecurity that we formerly lived in. In that case healing from the past is often needed to be able to live in the present without being driven by an illegitimate fear of our future.

Sally would be overcome with terror when anything happened that was out of the normal routine of things. She always pictured the worst case scenarios and couldn't stop herself. It became apparent she was being transported back to an earlier time when as a child there was no security or safe place in the midst of the chaos of her original alcoholic family. In many alcoholic homes, living with the fear and uncertainty of what might happen next *seemed* like normal life. However, it was not normal, it was terrifying and it deeply scared those living under it.

For many of us, the enemy of our souls has used our imaginations for his purposes and far too often we have just learned to shut it down in order to avoid the pictures. Our imaginations are necessary to feed our hearts and to be able to see and feel the Scriptures. To be healthy and live in peace, we need both our hearts and our minds flowing together in harmony along with our spirits that are connected to God's Spirit. Many Christians have just denied their fearful emotions by putting a lid on them, thereby deadening their hearts.

They then too often hide in their spirits while denying the emotions of the heart and sadly become without substance, since they are no longer connected even to themselves. I'm sure we have all met those who are so super-spiritual that we are unable to connect with them in any meaningful way and their spirituality never seems to feel very authentic. In that case, they are not connected in spirit, soul, and body, but separated within. For far too many years, I felt like the feather in the movie Forest Gump, floating here and there but having no substance. For me, one of the blessings of my healing has been to finally feel solid, connected, and anchored.

Many years ago I was one of those who lived in the denial of my real self. On some level of my heart, I considered real life to be emotionally scary and unacceptable. Unfortunately though, my feelings would always seem to leak out in unhealthy ways so I basically had no control over them. It wasn't until I finally faced the emotional fear and pain from the past I had buried and began healing, that I was able to begin to make good choices regarding how to handle my feelings. God made us with emotions, and since true life comes from the heart, our imaginations can feed our hearts for either good or bad.

CHAPTER 7

True Scriptural Pictures:
Using Our Imaginations Well

Pictures are the language of the heart, not just the mind. Our imagination is key to how we feed our hearts. Take the Scriptures for example, do you just read the words on the page or do you picture the words? Do you see the situation, feel what the people felt, connect with them when you experience some of those same emotions even though your particular circumstances might look very different? Do you hear Jesus talking to you personally through them? *"Taste and see The Lord is good."* (Psalm 34:8) We need to eat the Scriptures, not just read them. Enter them, connect with them instead of just gleaning information. Because I minister to people on the level of the heart with pictures, I recently overheard a person I had just counseled tell a friend, "She just made Jesus so real to me, I could feel him in a whole new way!" Jesus is real like that, but sometimes we have become so familiar with the stories that we read them intellectually, but do not enter them and experience them intimately with him on a heart level.

For example, let's really see Jesus as the good Shepherd who cares for his sheep (Psalm 23). *"I am your good Shepherd so you shall not be in want"* (my paraphrase). Picture that in whatever circumstances you find yourself right now. Do you feel lost, forsaken and alone, trapped in your situation? The good Shepherd looks after his sheep – he leaves the 99 in the care of the under-shepherd to find the one who feels trapped, lost, and alone, and who feels helpless and afraid. (Luke 15:3-6). Jesus our good Shepherd came to seek and save that one who is lost. His seeking us out is not just for salvation alone, but in whatever situation we find ourselves with those lost and alone feelings. He is looking for us and knocking on our heart's door. Allow your imagination to help you to see him come after you, feel his love as he picks you up and places you on his shoulder, close to his heart. Allow yourself to experience his strong, warm arms wrapping securely around you, supporting you and your weighty burden. (Isaiah 40:11)

A number of years ago as I was just beginning my honestly faced, authentic journey with Jesus (even though I had already known and walked with him for at least 25 years at that point), I found myself feeling like I was just beginning to walk with him as a very little child. I was, to use my little girl word *"ascared"*, having no clue as to how to do life, and feeling like I was about two years old. It was at that point I had a vision of a very winding path with Florida jungle on both sides. You know, the type of growth you can easily get caught in. Jesus was on the path and he sweetly said to me as the little two-year old, *"Hold my hand"*. I did that for a moment, but as two-year-olds are prone to do, I would drop his hand and find myself trapped and lost in the jungle by the side of the path. I would suddenly feel the horrible fear in the pit of my stomach of being lost and I'd frantically yell out for Jesus to find me. He would leave the path, look for me, then gently pick me up and bring me back to the roadway. He never scolded or rebuked me, but simply said with a kind smile, *"Hold my hand, I am the way"*. This happened over and over until I finally learned to hold onto his hand. Then I would look ahead at the path winding around the next curve and realize with terror that I couldn't see what was coming. What might be lurking there to hurt me? Jesus, aware of my terror and hesitancy, would lovingly repeat, "I am the way, just hold onto my hand".

I went through this scenario for three months before I was finally able to begin to trust him enough to truly enter the journey of learning to walk with him in rest. Then a new teaching began when he said, *"I am the truth"*. That took more months as I had to recognize the many lies I had believed. I had just accepted as truth my perceptions that were indeed, falsehood. By the end of that year, I was finally able to begin to learn what he meant when he repeatedly, still very kindly, told me, *"I am your life"*. The whole process

CHAPTER 7

took over a year, but trust finally began to grow in my heart as we walked together in those pictures. I am still daily walking that out on even deeper and deeper levels of my heart. The new foundation for my walk with Jesus was laid in that year.

There was another scriptural picture God gave me that has been truly significant in my healing and growth and I so share it with you that you also might find your specific place. You see, one of my early struggles had been that I always felt I had no place to belong – not in family, with friends, or in the church. I just didn't seem to fit. Jesus understood my struggle because he also had no place. Jesus in Luke 9:58 says, *"Foxes have holes and birds of the air have nests, but the Son of Man has no place to lay his head."*

The Spirit then showed me a very long table laden with all sorts of delights. People sitting in chairs surrounded this table that went on and on until I couldn't see it anymore, and there was smiling Jesus sitting at the head. He said to me, *"I have prepared a place for you, take the rightful place that I have paid for with my own body and blood. No one else can have that place for it has your name on it, so it's yours. But if you refuse to take it though through false unworthiness or shame, it will remain empty."* Then Jesus' countenance became increasingly sad as he said the last part. It had cost him his very life in order for me to have that seat. I began realize, as I finally took my place, that I had, unconsciously, pulled my chair back from the table just a little. Immediately my eyes were opened to see, that even though I had come to the table, I didn't see myself with value. Then Jesus told me these words, *"You are worth just as much as every one of my other children – no more, no less! Come take the place I have prepared for you from the foundation of the world."*

"In my Father's house are many rooms; if it were not so, I would have told you. I am going there to prepare a place for you." (John 14:2)

CHAPTER 8
Our Cooperation with God in Becoming Who We Were Designed to Be

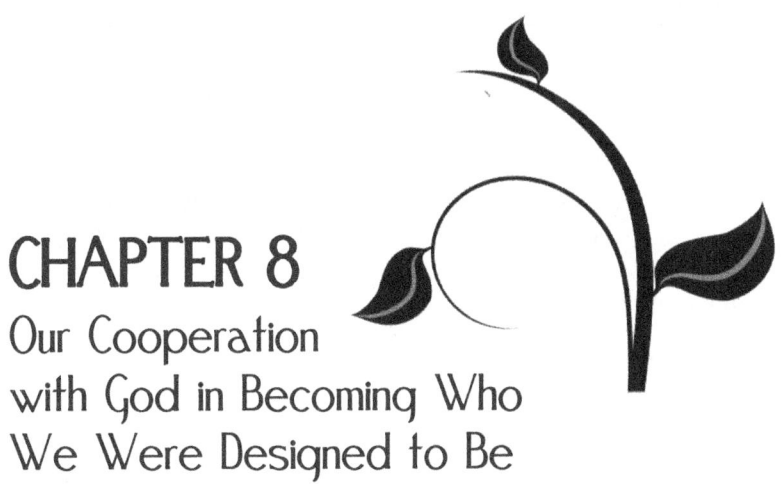

How do we cooperate with God in discovering our true selves? He is truly the only one who fully knows us and, as the scriptures remind us, he knew us before we were ever born, for it was from the womb he called and named us. (Psalm 139 & Isaiah 49) Imagine this... God knew us before our parents did! He received us from birth and has been longing to share with us who he has always known and seen us to be... (Psalm 71:6 & Psalm 27:10). Our souls are the seat of our mind, will, and emotions and have been wounded through our past emotional pain. At the core of my being, influencing my emotions, I secretly believed I was a throwaway, just like a piece of garbage! Until we have healing in our souls, others, as well as ourselves, usually have never even met the real "us" – we have only revealed what we determined the acceptable parts because the rest has been buried in shame. (Romans 12:9) Too much of my early life had been spent as a chameleon changing into whoever anyone wanted me to be. My unspoken cry was, "Please accept me, don't throw me away!"

You know how it is when you see things in someone, maybe even one of your children – buried treasures that they have never seen for themselves. It's incredibly sad when you see them sabotage themselves over and over, because without their realizing it, they are living out of a self-protective survival system they have erected to do life instead of from who they really are created to be. If God really knows us as well as the Bible says, then the logical thing is to bring the questions about who we really are to him. Many ask him that question, but in a haphazard, superficial manner. Instead, we need be focused to actually mine for the treasure we are and commit to do whatever is necessary to find the answer. It can sometimes take much time and effort to discover the real self that lies hidden under the self-protective false structures that have been built early in life just to survive, but it's well worth it. You will love being the real you! I hear that all the time from the people I am working with who have been willing to pursue their true selves.

Questions to Ask Yourself

- *How do you think about and speak to yourself?*
- *Does your self-talk reflect care and consideration or is it laced with self-contempt and anger?*
- *Do you angrily react to the difficult circumstances that God allows and do you recognize those reactions as reflective of some possible false beliefs about God?*
- *Do you blame yourself, others, or perhaps life itself?*
- *Do you take time to be with yourself or do you constantly drown out your desires and escape from yourself, perhaps using Facebook, internet games, TV?*
- *What do you love – do you even know?*
- *Have you even taken the time to even ponder and explore?*
- *Do you pay attention to your heart, or are you living from your head alone?*
- *Are there wounds from your past that have scabbed over, but still contain an infection of sorts, and were never truly healed? If so, why?*

- *Are you worth whatever it might take to heal from the past? Do you tend to live in the past and/or fear the future, ignoring or missing the present?*

I did that for years, I was always reacting from the past or fearing the future, but sadly missed the enjoyment of the present moment. Working with God in healing the hurts of our past gives us the ability to be fully alive in the present with joyful anticipation toward our future.

Those are just a few of the signs that we have not fully taken the time to really know ourselves. How do you get to know someone you have just met? If the relationship is going to be more than a superficial one, you will start to tell each other your stories, you will ask questions with interest and care about the other person, and begin to connect with them on a heart level. It takes time to build real relationships; the Bible warns about ones that are built quickly because they usually don't last. Just like a tree has to have a healthy root system in order to be strong, the tree that quickly grows up without it, just as quickly can become top-heavy and be blown down. What if you were to spend some time and effort into getting to know the real you? Who might you find? One thing you would find is a heart with wonderful treasures as well as it's having broken places. I have been doing pastoral counseling for well over thirty years and I have never seen a heart I haven't loved. I haven't always liked the covering mask or survival system the person projected, but as I would get glimpses of who they really were, it became apparent their real heart was wonderful and worth digging for.

Once again, I ask... *what do you love, what brings you life when you do it, what lights you up and exhilarates you? If you were to list all the various things that do, what is it about those things that you like? What do they have in common?* Usually we notice no common denominator at a surface glance because they might seem to be unrelated, but they often have a common theme.

CHAPTER 8

Let me give you an example from the life of someone I met with just last week. I was asking him those questions and he shared a few things he loved like snowboarding, surfing, being in business for himself, enjoying what was not a nine to five job, and a few things in other areas. I knew a bit of his early background that had included some control that had inflicted pain, so I could immediately see a common dominator. What I observed was that if he was to live the life he was created for and experience the joy of more fully living his own life, it had to include *freedom!* Everything he loved included freedom, not foolish, selfish freedom, but because he has an adventurous spirit and is a creative person, the need for the freedom to release his life and creativity was paramount. When we know what we're about on a deep heart level, we can make easier choices regarding career, ministry, or most anything because whatever brings us real life must include that specific thing.

I'll give you another example from my own life. I never had much of any guidance in my life and felt lost for far too many years, not knowing who I was. After going on this journey to find my own heart and life, and discovering what God had put into me way back when I was created, I began to recognize what it was I loved to do. As an unfortunate result, I was always searching for that perfect place to do it. Did I want to counsel, teach, do groups, lead Bible studies, write – what? As I kept asking God about it, he asked me, "What is your call?" As I pondered that, I realized the thing that drives me on the deepest level of my heart is to see captives freed to be who they are created to be.

The scriptures that God gave me 35 years ago, far before I had any clue about what they even meant, laid out my call. That call was to co-labor with Jesus in seeing captives go free and then working with him to remove the obstacles that kept his people trapped in their own prisons. If that was truly my call, then it doesn't really matter how it plays out. It could be in Starbucks over a cup of coffee, sharing before a crowd at a church meeting, one on one counseling, writing a book like this, in an email, running into an old friend in the supermarket, wherever. Unconsciously, even at a party, I find myself listening and sharing with someone the Lord puts in my path. Whatever I do, and I do it all day long, but not as ministry, simply because that's what I'm made to do – so it's not work, but joy! Just recently, overhearing me talk to someone at a dinner party, I was jokingly asked, "Aren't you ever off the clock?" The answer to that is, no, because that's what I'm all about!

What are you about? What drives you, not as a work, but as joy? What are some of the ways it plays out? I'm not talking about escapes though. There are many things we think we love and do enjoy on some level, but they have often been just ways to escape from life when it gets too difficult. I don't know how many men (usually more than women, but women have other escapes like shopping) that have loved video games. Yet even in video games, there can be a clue of something they are not finding in everyday life that touches on some elements of who they were created to be. We are created for adventure, but if we escape from the adventure of being present in our real lives, we often find other outlets. What can we learn from even the things we might escape into – what might they be providing for us as a substitute for our really living life?

One young guy in particular comes to mind who was pretty much addicted. When I asked him to ponder deeply on what playing certain video games gave him, a sense of adventure came to the surface. In his everyday life, he was feeling trapped in duty and dullness, but in the game it was a different story. Maybe not in his real life, but there he could enter into many battles and try to win! It gave him opportunity for power, when in real life he was experiencing powerlessness and frustration! If we are created for adventure, and when we just settle for existence, we often have to look for vicarious ways to experience that desire.

However, then we are not really living our own life the way we were meant to. We are simply escaping through a substitute, sometimes even dangerous ones. Our lives are meant to be filled with the adventure of co-laboring with Jesus. On a day to day basis we each co-labor in our own unique way, with our own particular giftings, within our own given sphere of influence.

Understanding the Times and Seasons of Our Lives

Ecclesiastes 3:1-8
"There is a time for everything, and a season for every activity under heaven; a time to be born and a time to die, a time to plant and a time to uproot, a time to kill and a time to heal, a time to tear down and a time to build; a time to weep and a time to laugh, a time to mourn and a time to dance, a time to scatter stones and a time to gather them, a time to embrace and a time to refrain, a time to search and a time to give up, a time to keep and a time to throw away, a time to tear and a time to mend, a time to be silent and a time to speak, a time to love and a time to hate, a time for war and a time for peace."

Jesus said in the end of Matthew 16:3, *"...You know how to interpret the appearance of the sky, but you cannot interpret the signs of the times."* Understanding times and seasons is so important for our lives in order to cooperate with what God is doing at any particular *time*. It's like hitting our head against the wall when we are trying to do the right thing in the wrong season. We might have an accurate prophetic word from God, but yet we don't see it come to pass because it's not yet the right season. Over and over throughout the Bible, we see phrases like, *"In the fullness of time..."*, *"When the time had fully come..."*, etc. Even in referring to his death, Jesus said at one point that his time had not yet come. Jesus only did what he saw and heard his Father doing. As we grow in intimacy with him, we begin to hear his voice more accurately which is of utmost importance or we will become out of sync and discouraged.

Two Winds

I just recently came across a prophetic word that was nationally given in 1987. At the time I read it, I knew it to be truth and through all the years since, I have never been able to forget it. As it was once again put into my hands, I realized that we are now beginning to live in the season prophesied so it brought even more clarity to the current time. The prophecy spoke of two winds. One wind would look like it was bringing devastation but it would only shake that which needed to be shaken. The name of that wind was, *"Holiness Unto The Lord"*, and God said it was his wind. Those who were willing to put their face in that wind and allow God to change them would be prepared for the second wind that was coming – that wind was called, *"The Kingdom of God"*. That wind would bring in God's government and order as well as supernatural power. It would bring forth his harvest and what God was desiring to do on the earth. When I first received a copy of that prophecy I knew it to be true, but back then I didn't see it happening. However, as I recently saw it again, I realized the time was now upon us.

We all have different seasons that we go through at various times. To understand the bigger picture of what God is doing with us at any given period, it is helpful to recognize our present season. That is so important if we are to cooperate with him and not get discouraged. Just as in nature, our seasons will change, so if it's your winter, there is always hope that spring will finally break forth. Recognizing whether you are in an exciting spring season with wonderful shoots of green growth and revelation, or a pleasant summertime of rest and simply walking with Jesus quietly in the garden, can help us to cooperate with what he is doing. Perhaps you are presently in an amazing harvest season where many of the seeds you have planted in the spring are finally maturing.

However the most difficult season of all to endure can be our winter season. At that time everything, as well as ourselves, can appear to be lifeless, without growth – fruitless. It feels cold, dull, gray, and without energy and purpose, and maybe even like winter in Alaska – dark. Isaiah 45:3 promises, *"I will give you the treasures of the darkness, riches stored in secret places so that you may know that I am The Lord, the God of Israel, who summons you by name."* Many treasures come forth from that dark, barren season, and even when it appears like nothing is happening, God is working deep within us. Far more truly deep growth within us comes out of an extended winter season than often happens in other seasons. When I see someone after they have gone through one of their most difficult winter seasons, I am often amazed at the new growth that is bursting forth, new shoots of revelation and deep heart change that then makes the way for spring to come with new life. It was through one of my most difficult, dark winter seasons that I learned to finally begin to deeply trust God.

When I see someone in their winter season, I am always reminded of a winter tree up north. We had many such trees behind our house in New Jersey, that throughout the winter appeared to be dead, but they were actually being strengthened by the harsh winds and cold temperatures. As I looked out of my kitchen window, it was difficult to believe they would ever be full of life again. But one day... those tiny green buds began to burst forth, and then almost overnight the trees were transformed! What beauty to behold – life full of splendor once again returned!

In certain seasons, even our quiet times with God can begin to feel dull and dutiful instead of life-giving. When people go through a season like that, I often ask them what feels more alive? Sometimes it will be just listening to worship music or quietly sitting with God outside in his creation. In those times, sometimes the Bible can begin to feel dull, and prayer seems to be just hitting the ceiling. Too often what happens next is they either give up on it all or guilt themselves into going through the motions. Particularly, when a person is going through some deep emotional healing, even church can feel like it's a difficult place to be. I've had many tell me that, but as the heaviness in them lifted, new understanding and time of refreshment took its place. So that is not just a time to guilt yourself or escape, but you might find you have to meet with God in a whole new honest, non-religious way.

That's a good time to really look at the wonder of God's creation and meet with him there. Let the Spirit show you his handiwork in the sky, the trees – go to the beach if that feeds your soul. Just talk with him and share your thoughts, dreams, disappointments, and fears. Jesus has also experienced those things as a man and he's your best counselor, there with you 24/7. It's also a good time to write from your heart, but do more than journal, write a personal letter to Jesus, expressing the things that you might not share with anyone else.

He knows your struggles and even any anger or disappointment you might have toward him. He desires to share with you and have fellowship with you in your suffering, because he walked this earth and understands! It is also an opportunity to develop a thankful heart, looking for those tiny things that bring blessing even among the losses. Developing a thankful heart is one of the most important things we can do with God and for ourselves in any season. It transforms us from a complainer to a worshipper in all circumstances! (1 Thessalonians 5:16-18) *"Rejoice always, pray continually, give thanks in all circumstances; for this is God's will for you in Christ Jesus."* We don't worship *for the circumstances*, but we worship God *over* them.

The season of finding our true selves can at times seem very long and so it's natural to feel weary, but developing a thankful heart on the journey is one of the most important things we can do. In the Old Testament God's people in the wilderness went through a lot because of their grumbling. When we are in a winter or wilderness season, it can far too often feel unending and since we don't really understand what is happening to us, it feels very natural to complain. After all, "Where is God anyway?" "Why did he leave me here and seemingly just disappear?" After honestly sharing our struggle with him, it is helpful to move toward developing a heart of thanksgiving and praise acknowledging that God does know what's going on, and that he does have us in the palm of his hand even when it doesn't seem that way.

In a particular season of my own struggle, and after pages of writing out my angst, my fears, in my letter to God, he answered me with: *"My child, my ways are good and healing and right. Even though you don't yet understand. I know the paths seem rocky at times and the uprooting is hard and slow. Come to me and rest. I am building you and your life in a way the gates of hell cannot shake. All this is part of your journey of Life with me, in me, and through me. Come. We will live, move, and have our being together so you are never alone. Come. Rest, trust, hold tightly to me. I will unfold your journey of life, not death. Resurrection life is being birthed in you so it can then flow out to others. I will take even your messes and work them together for good as you allow me. I am right here in your midst and I have never left you, nor will I ever."*

Learning to Abide

Abiding, resting, remaining in him is what Jesus longs for with us. We see that spelled out for us in John 15 as Jesus begins that wonderful chapter on abiding with the picture of the vine and branches. When we remain stuck with our hearts shut down in fear or anger toward God or others, we are like the branch that is no longer connected to the tree. Before long it withers and dies without the sap of life flowing into it. As our vital heart connection with Jesus closes down through separation, we become angry, ungrateful, uncaring, judgmental blamers. Our ability to love has been affected much like when someone steps on a garden hose causing the flow to become just a trickle.

We are just clay, flesh, intellect without Jesus' breath of life. Jesus is not far off – his Spirit lives within us so he is closer to us than our breath, but how often we simply neglect and lose our own hearts in the busyness of life with the sad result that we no longer even sense his presence within. The reality though is that Jesus is still there waiting inside us, however we have cut off the source of the true life that comes from him. We might produce much and be acclaimed and admired by many, yet still be disconnected from the life source within. No wonder we so easily stress and burn out for once we begin to live on our own again, we are moving away from the only source of true life. God doesn't disconnect from our hearts, we do!

For years I went in and out of that. I would get angry at God's inactivity in something important to me and without realizing it, I would disconnect, simply like hanging up the phone! Then I would feel all alone in my world and begin stressing over small stuff. It wasn't long then until I wanted to begin to control my life again.

I find far too many Christians are like spiritual leap frogs! I know I was like that for many years, jumping in and out. Into the flow of real life and connection with him – out to doing things on my own again and into stagnation. In a spiritual environment, good worship, or prayer time, it is easy to connect back with your heart, but then as "life" happens, there is a disconnect and duty too often begins to take over! You might check in at the beginning or the end of the day, but

CHAPTER 8

what happens in between? Do you flow with him, listen to him, bring him into the decisions, and stay tuned to anytime he "checks" you within? Are you being led by the grace and peace of Jesus from within, or perhaps, you not even aware of it?

Another place we can disconnect is when we look at our calendars and see what either is, or is not, looming ahead. For years I got ahead of myself by struggling with, "How can I do it all?" or on the opposite side, "The days are too empty!" Anxiety would be birthed and pressure to handle it all would creep in. As I increasingly learned to abide, I began to recognize that God was already ahead of me and would either give me the grace to endure or cause my circumstances to change.

As I am finally learning to allow God to take over my calendar, it's amazing how often he rearranges it with cancellations. At the same time, waiting in the wings, is the one who desperately needs that appointment! Just this week, with flu season in full swing, as I entered the office, someone said to me, "If anyone gets the flu and you get a cancellation, I need the appointment". Little did she know that, just before I left home, I received a cancellation from someone with the flu!

Abiding takes us back to the internal rest of the Garden where life was stress free, full of joy, and peaceful. Since toiling with all its pressure and sweat came in after the Fall of man and was part of the curse, simply tending the particular garden we were designed for is meant to bring delight, fulfillment, and joy. Sure there are stressors because we still live in a broken world, but how we react and handle them depends largely on whether or not we are abiding in him and seeing him in everything that comes across our path.

If he is there right in the midst with us in even the hard things that happen, the unfair things, the hurtful, and the stressful things, we are not left on our own to handle them. If the Spirit truly wants to walk through the deep waters with us and promises we won't drown in the process, he is also the way through so we have someone to lean on and rest in, even in our discomfort and confusion. Unfortunately though, with every new, difficult circumstance we often have to wrestle through to be able to rest again, however the more history of his faithfulness we have experienced, the easier it becomes.

"When you pass through the waters, I will be with you; and when you pass through the rivers, they will not sweep over you. When you walk through the fire, you will not be burned; the flames will not set you ablaze. For I am The Lord your God, the Holy One of Israel, your Savior;..." (Isaiah 43:2,3a)

God designed each of us with uniqueness, with a creativity far too many of us have never fully discovered! He has given us gifts that are meant to be released that will bring us deep satisfaction, but only as we flow from that Source of Life within us whose name is Jesus. Recently, as I was praying about the things that were on my plate for the day and two of the people I had been quite concerned about, the Lord spoke to me as I was writing my letter to him that morning.

He said, *"Abide in me – it's about openness not awareness. If you remain in me and allow me room to flow with you, then we move together in harmony. Out of that combined union of our beings, rivers of living water are released to those around you even without your awareness. I am outside of time so the time factor is not a problem. I can bring back words to people from years ago, even when you are sleeping! For I sleep not."*

"He who dwells (abides) in the shelter of the Most High, will rest in the shadow of the Almighty" (Psalm 91:1). The Amplified Bible states the result of our dwelling in him will be so we remain stable and fixed. Verse 2 in the Amplified, *"...He is my Refuge and my Fortress, my God; on him I lean and*

CHAPTER 8

rely and in him I (confidently) trust". To abide means that we must release our control and risk trusting him in deeper ways than we possibly ever have before.

It requires an intimacy with him; learning to hear his still small voice within and saying a wholehearted, willing "yes" to the things he asks of us. It is very similar to how a small child responds to a loving parent with simple heart-felt obedience, often without understanding why because they simply trust in the parent's good heart toward them. Picture a loving mother or father with a small child here – the little one trusting, resting in the parent's safe, caring arms or taking their hand and walking into the unknown. It's enough that the parent knows the way.

"Remain (abide, stay) in me and I will remain in you. No branch can bear fruit by itself; it must remain in the vine. Neither can you bear fruit unless you remain in me." (John 15:4). The Amplified Bible translates abide as dwell. *"Dwell in me and I will dwell in you."* Many of us might have known these scriptures for years on a head level and truly believed they were spiritual truths. However learning to actually abide, remain, dwell, stay connected to our hearts moment by moment when all is crumbling around us is a very different thing.

"I am the Vine; you are the branches. Whoever lives in me and I in him will bear much fruit. However apart from me (cut off from vital union with me) you can do nothing." (John 15:5) Do you get the picture how important it is that we don't jump in and out of the life of Jesus within us, but remain connected, continually living our lives from that center? (Acts 17:28) *"For in him we live and move and have our being."* The sad reality here is that when we disconnect from our own hearts, we have ceased to abide in him and are back to living life on our own!

Jesus desires to walk in that kind of unity of heart and flow with us – harmony and trusting rest in him no matter what might be happening around us. (Isaiah 32:18-20) *"My people will live in peaceful dwelling places, in secure homes, in undisturbed places of rest though hail flattens the forest and the city is leveled completely; how blessed you will be sowing your seed by every stream, and letting your cattle and donkeys range free."* It's only through getting to know Jesus that intimately and through learning to abide in him with childlike trust that the above is possible.

Jesus told us that if we are willing to become as little children, we can begin to see his kingdom in the midst of a world that is crumbling around us. I believe these are the days of preparation for whatever might be down the road. For each of us it might take a willingness to wrestle through with our faith to finally be able to come to that kind of resting and abiding place in him.

Abiding also involves a dying to ourselves with all our selfishness and sometimes quiet willfulness that demands to have things go our own way. However, I have also seen far too many Christians, without healthy boundaries, pour out their lives for the selfishness of others. As a result, they sadly become burned out and used by people in very unhealthy ways, all in the name of Christianity. That is not God's way, so it is imperative we have learned personal boundaries and have clear discernment from the Spirit. However, the more we have learned to listen and abide in Jesus, the quicker we sense the internal check when someone is trying to use, control, or take advantage. Jesus was never led by people; he only did what he saw his Father doing. So must we.

Jesus' last prayer for his disciples, as he poured out his heart to God before facing the cross alone, included us (John 17:20). He longed in prayer for the unity we would experience with he and his Father and that we would be *one* just as they are *united* in the Trinity. (John 17). True unity,

CHAPTER 8

that level of belonging and resting comes out of our learning to abide in him on a continual basis, no longer jumping in and out of his life within us. Our lives are meant to be lived from an open, connected heart, communing with him even in the midst of our activity-crowded lives. Too often though, people tell me, "I'm too busy now, I'll talk to God later about that." Without realizing it, they are abandoning their unity with him to handle things on their own. Sometimes we wrongly see prayer as something we do. Instead it is "our breath" that we breathe out to him from a heart that is open and in union with Jesus.

This is not something we learn quickly any more than keeping our hearts from closing over is easily learned. One major reason for our hearts closing over is the wall of self-protection we have erected around it. Experiencing hurt over and over throughout our lives often causes us to take matters into our own hands. We place a cover over our hearts so it becomes much easier and safer to live from our intellects and outside of our hearts. That might work to keep us feeling safer, but also it prevents us from truly loving ourselves or others deeply from the heart. It also prevents us from truly trusting God.

In Paul's letter to the Corinthians, he urged them several times to *open wide their hearts*. We can grasp many truths but still be far from experientially living them out. Without even realizing it, we can lead self-protected lives with our hearts closed off, longing for real life, but missing it completely. *"Keep and guard your heart with all vigilance and above all that you guard, for out of it flow the springs of life."* (Proverbs 4:23 AMP). Then Jesus said, *"He who believes in Me [who cleaves to and trusts in and relies on Me] as the Scripture has said, from his innermost being shall flow [continuously] springs and rivers of living water"* (John 7:38 AMP). Jesus reminds us that streams of living water are simply meant to flow out to the world around us from our innermost being. But our being must remain connected in unity with God.

When we enter the flow from his heart that is connected to our hearts, it is easy.

Abiding doesn't come first from the head, but from the heart, and then as our head understands more fully, it connects with our heart in unity – not the other way around. That creates a flow, a harmony and unity within us that even begins to bring well-being to our bodies. Therefore, healing can begin to be released from the inside out. The first unity that actually has to happen is a unity within ourselves (Psalm 86:11b *"...give me an undivided heart that I may fear your name"*). From an undivided heart there can begin a wonderful unity with the heart of the Godhead that easily overflows out from us as a river.

As we each flow with God' Spirit from the unity within us, true unity can begin in the Body. That unity within us allows us to begin participating with God in greater measure than ever before, releasing a life-giving flow to others. Are you a life-giver to those you come in contact with? If not yet, do you desire to be? The Spirit of Jesus desires to co-labor with us in our own uniqueness to reach people who have been lost, hurting, and wounded. That flow pours out of an undivided, committed, and surrendered heart even without our awareness. It is exciting when others later thank you for something you didn't even know you did or said!

The ability to surrender our will and hurts to him more fully comes out of that undivided heart as well. In Psalm 51, David asks God to create a *"willing heart"* within him, and in Philippians 2:12b-13 we read, *"continue to work out your salvation with fear and trembling, for it is God who works in you to will and to act according to his good purpose."* With that surrendered heart, we more easily begin to be able to recognize our own tendencies toward willfulness and the selfish demanding of our own ways. We begin to see motivations we might never have recognized before.

CHAPTER 8

A spirit of repentance begins to grow within us – repentance not just for sins we have committed, but for our whole willful nature that has far too many times, simply wanted to do things our own way. (Isaiah 53 *"We each like sheep, have gone astray, each of us has turned to his own way..."*) Our desires and purposes begin to line up with his, not the other way around.

It has been my experience that the emotions of peace and rest flooding my soul reveal to me that I have surrendered from my heart. I have learned that if there is not peace, there has not been full heart surrender, perhaps surrender in the mind, but not yet in my heart.

CHAPTER 9
Learning to Live with Peace in a World of Turmoil and Uncertainty

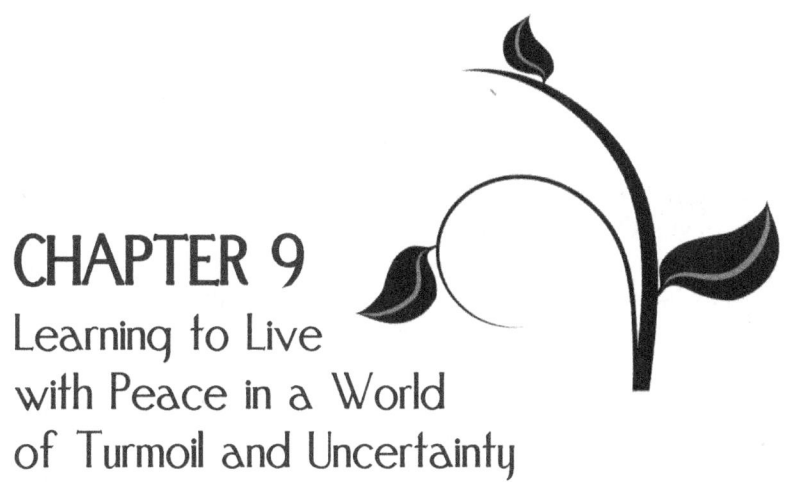

A very brief glance at the world around us reveals the unsettling times we live in – there is no longer any way to pretend otherwise unless we choose to live in total denial. Nature seems almost out of control with floods, tornados, hurricanes, tidal waves, wild fires, not to mention the wars and rumors of wars as well as the lurking threat of terrorism all over the world. It seems like every major area is in crisis – governmental, financial, medical, educational to name just a few. In our country alone, one tragedy ends and another too quickly begins with just about every state affected. So how do we live from a place of peace, not denial, in the midst of such turmoil? More and more voices are proclaiming that we are living in the end times, but of course the period known as the end times could be very lengthy. If that is the case, how do we then continue to live with peace?

Strangely, I believe God is training us to learn to trust him as our only true security through many of the personal struggles we are going through. It's so easy to look for man or government to save us, but another glance tells us the whole world system is in danger and our only hope of real long-term security is in God. *"He will be the sure foundation for your times, a rich store of salvation and wisdom and knowledge; the fear of The Lord is the key to this treasure."* (Isaiah 33:6) Verses like that are easy to believe with our intellects and to speak out of our mouths, but when difficult personal times invade our lives, what do our emotions and behaviors tell us about our true level of trust? Jesus said we will know where we really are by our fruit so what happens to us internally when trouble hits? What is the fruit our lives show forth? Peace? Angst? Fear? How are we really feeling on the deepest level of our hearts? Is there a strange peace there even while we are struggling, or is there a silent terror? Our anxiety might be telling a different story than the one we are speaking out of our mouths.

I believe a key scripture that gives us a bigger picture and understanding of the shaking going on in many of our lives right now is from Jeremiah 31:28. *"Just as I watched over them to uproot and tear down and to overthrow, destroy and bring disaster so I will watch over them to build and to plant', declares The Lord."* Notice there are five things describing the process of uprooting our survival systems and false pictures, but they are all done in order to build us back up on the right foundation of God alone. Then he is able to plant us where each of us belongs. Remember Jesus' words that a house built on a bad foundation will eventually crumble when the torrents (or circumstances) come. He is rebuilding us on the Rock that is Christ Jesus himself and that will never crumble no matter what happens around us!

One thing God seems to be breaking concerns our false pictures of security. Somehow the American dream has far too often gotten mixed up with it all. That, along with the spirit of entitlement that too often says we *deserve* our lives to look a certain way and to work for us because we should be able to be happy. How many times we have quietly demanded to know our future instead of, even without understanding, entrusting our futures to a good and caring God. Many I've worked with, who have allowed God to begin to heal their wounded hearts, have shared with me the new discovery that now as trouble comes to them personally, even though they feel disturbed, a strange peace is also there. That peace is still small but increasingly growing within them even though they still feel a little afraid.

Looking at peace from the whole of scripture, gives us a much deeper understanding than we might have had in the past. *Completeness, wholeness, health, welfare, safety, soundness, tranquility, prosperity, perfectness, fullness, rest, harmony, absence of agitation or discord* are some of the ways it's described. Jesus is the Prince of Peace and since he is pleased to dwell within us by his Spirit, we have all of the above available to us, no matter what the circumstances, as we learn to abide and draw from his life and peace within us.

A respected prophetic voice said that Proverbs 3:5,6 was one of the most valuable scriptures for us to really grasp for the times that lay ahead. *"Trust in The Lord with all your heart and lean not on your own understanding; in all your ways acknowledge him, and he will make your paths straight."* All that is easier said than done however, and it is usually a long struggle for each of us to learn how to rest and trust in the midst of our own personal adversity. Not to mention what is lurking in the bigger picture of world's problems. However, the more we develop a history of trust with God in our personal stories, we will be able to become increasingly peaceful in the larger world story that is unfolding all around us, even though the darkness is getting darker. In our adversity, if we allow his Spirit to teach us how to trust him with our personal stories, it can enable us to become more restful in him and his ways in the larger picture of life.

"When you pass through the waters, I will be with you; and when you pass through the rivers, they will not sweep over you. When you walk through the fire, you will not be burned; the flames will not set you ablaze. For I am The Lord your God, the Holy One of Israel, your Savior...". (Isaiah 43:2-3)

CHAPTER 9

"'For my thoughts are not your thoughts, neither are your ways my ways', declares The Lord. 'As the heavens are higher than the earth, so are my ways higher than your ways and my thoughts than your thoughts.'" (Isaiah 55:8,9)

"The fruit of that righteousness will be peace; its effect will be quietness and confidence forever. My people will live in peaceful dwelling places, in secure homes, in undisturbed places of rest. Though hail flattens the forest and the city is leveled completely, how blessed you will be, sowing your seed by every stream, and letting your cattle and donkeys range free." (Isaiah 32:17-20)

The Bigger Picture of Our Lives

We are created for far more than pleasure and enjoyment, but for what? I believe God is equipping, whosoever will, to co-labor with him in a far bigger story than we could have ever imagined, but it will look different for each of us. Living our true story will however, bring us deep satisfaction and pleasure. Unfortunately, the way we have thought life should look has to break in order to be able to see higher and walk with Jesus in his ways. Too often, prayer in past seasons has been spent in trying to get God to cooperate with our own thoughts and plans. We tried to bring him down to our way of thinking and doing things instead of allowing him to lift us higher to see his. We must be willing to wait as we sit with him in heavenly places, which then eventually opens our eyes to a view of his bigger picture. It's only when we begin to see a circumstance from his perspective and learn to cooperate with what he is doing, that a whole new way of living opens up to us. In Revelation 4, we hear the ascended Jesus saying, *"Come up here and I will show you what must take place after this."*

Just today I met with someone for the first time. As I often have to do, it was first necessary to open her eyes to a whole new way of viewing her life circumstances from God's perspective (the beginning of the story) instead of through her pain. She shared that it gave her a whole new starting place for healing from the hurts she experienced. Too often we come into the real story mid-way through.

Jesus "learned obedience from what he suffered", so could that be how we learn to walk with him in his ways as well? (Hebrews 5:8) Could it be that our personal struggles, whether they have been financial, relational, or whatever, have really been our teachers? (Isaiah 30:20-22) (John 5:19) *"Jesus gave them this answer: 'I tell you the truth, the Son can do nothing by himself, he can only do what he sees his Father doing, because whatever the Father does, the Son also does."* (John 15:4) Can we do any less in trying to live this life?

We are all made for adventure, but our love of comfort and false security has softened us. Believe me, I love my comfort more than most, but I keep sensing God has a far bigger plan than just our enjoyment of the American dream. I desire to be a part of what God is doing in the earth even though I'm more than mid-way through my seventies! There is a battle for real life raging whether we are aware of it or not. Up to this point much of it has been going on in the heavenlies, but we are now seeing it manifesting on the earth all around us. Will we just put our fingers in our ears and try to pretend all will be well, or will we begin to struggle with what we really believe, what our lives are really about, and begin to allow God to re-teach us his way of really living?

What is happening on the earth is bigger than we know. Each one of us is needed to become who we were intended to be before we experienced an identity theft by the enemy of our souls. Each one of us is needed. We see a lot of the stealing of people's identity in the natural, but there has been an even greater identity theft on the level of our inner being and purpose. It often began very early in our lives. Fighting for our true selves is of the utmost importance because it is

CHAPTER 9

opposed by the enemy and won't happen without our participation. We are each needed in our own unique way, but we usually cannot begin to see how until we find our true selves. God uniquely created each of us – on purpose for purpose – and has called every one of us into being for such a time in history as this.

Your life matters, so it is time to awaken, not to fear, but to become who you really are. Only the God who knew you before your parents did, knows who that is. It is time for each of us to discover our true security is in God and not in man or in his systems even though that sort of trust does not come quickly or easily. We are in a season of preparation for far greater purposes than we could imagine. The problem is that none of us can see clearly yet what it will all look like. The Bible just gives us glimpses.

In trying to live life beginning with our *own* understanding, a prayer I have unfortunately heard far too often has been, *"Tell me what to do God, and I'll do it"*. Unfortunately that is not usually how it works – God doesn't always tell us what to do, instead we learn to hear what he is doing in any given situation and join with *him* in *his* ways. That's what Jesus did. One of the most important verses of my life, in a very practical sense, has been Jesus speaking to me, *"I am the way..."*. I, very painfully and slowly, have had to learn (and am still daily learning) to walk with him step by step in trust instead of obtaining the knowledge of what exactly he is doing and where he is taking me.

Since knowledge can make us feel like we're in control, it feels much safer to try to understand than to simply trust him to lead us as a child is led along by a loving father. In that leading, I often feel clueless and have found God seldom gives me the full story. More often I get just a glimpse of the destination, and then he allows the journey to unfold one step at a time. As I take the first step, the next one often opens up, but sometimes there can be even a few steps and then a waiting... Just like with this book that took almost two years to complete. I can see that God is doing something big in the earth and that we each have a part to play, but I can't see the details of how it all plays out even for my own life. I'm sure that frustrates you as it does me, but it also increases our dependency on him for even the next step to take. If we remain yoked with him on the journey though, we truly discover what Jesus said to be true when he promised rest to us who were weary with the burden of life. (Matthew 11:28-30) We might even discover ourselves to be a part of something larger than we ever imagined!

After walking with Jesus for over forty-plus years, I am finally learning that real life consists of simply showing up for life each day with Jesus. I don't have to know what anything is going to look like or have any particular expectation, but simply join with him in whatever he unfolds. I am still learning to remain present with him in the moment, whatever that moment happens to look like. However, in order to do that in the midst of the mixture of a fallen world, separating the gifts from the losses can be crucial because, most of the time, there are both. As we accept that fact and grieve our losses with Jesus, our hearts begin to experience joy and thankfulness. I am learning that the more I stay present with that, the more I see my life as a shared adventure!

Below are God's words to me that I believe are for you as well on this amazingly wonderful, but sometimes difficult journey of life --yes they are true even in the midst of our struggles and mess-ups! Even when we feel clueless as to our next step and we are overwhelmed with the journey, he is *Jevohah Shammah*, the God who is always *THERE*, right in our midst never leaving or forsaking us.

"The Lord is there." (Ezekiel 48:35)

CHAPTER 9

"Never will I leave you, never will I forsake you." (Hebrews 13:5)

"My child, my ways are good and healing and right even though the paths are rocky at times and the uprooting process is hard and slow. Come to me and rest. I am building you and your life in a way the gates of hell cannot shake. All this is part of your Journey of Life in me, life that is really life. This dimension of living comes only through remaining in me. Come. We will live, move, and have our being together so you are never alone. Come, rest, trust, hold tightly to me and I will unfold your journey of true life. Resurrection life will be birthed out all that you are willing to 'die' to so my life can then flow through those things and they no longer hold you captive. As a result, true life is able flow within you and pour out of you to others even without your awareness. Yes, you have messed up and will continue to mess up at times, but trust me to work even your mess-up's together for good. I am now leading you, not only in the Way, but on the Highway of Holiness." (Isaiah 35)

Help me Lord... I am still a mess and a mess-up at times, but I long to walk with you in your holiness (wholeness) on that highway and bring true life and freedom to others. I desire that my life brings you glory. Only by remaining in you, can I do it. Thanks.

CHAPTER 10
Viewing Even Death from an Eternal Perspective

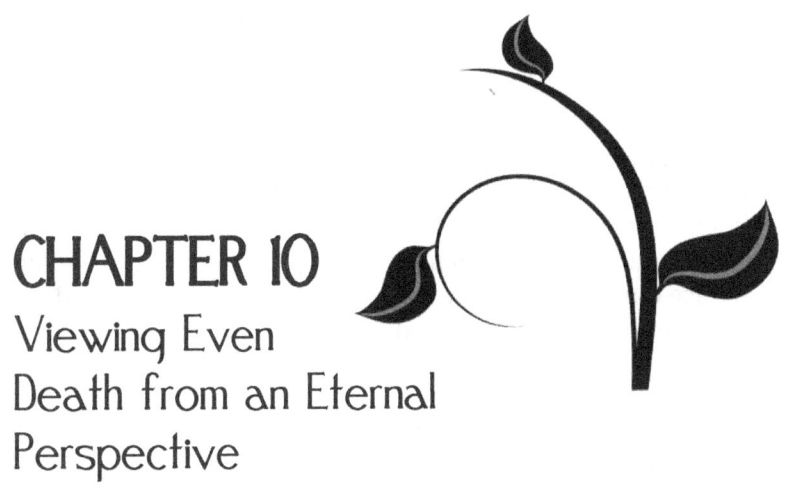

To live with passion and joy in the midst of a broken world, we must be able to see beyond our fears and struggles. We don't do that by ignoring or pushing them under the carpet. We face the reality of life as it is head on, and then we meet with Jesus there where he is waiting with arms open wide as our only true Rock and strong foundation. He longs to carry us through our stresses and have us join him in the even greater reality of what he is doing in the earth. He is patiently working in individuals, churches, nations, even in our own hearts and lives. As we grasp that fact and learn to cooperate with him, we can become a part of what he is doing on a far larger scale than we ever have before.

Jesus is a Redeemer, a Restorer, a Healer of broken hearts. He desires to take all the pain and sorrow we have experienced throughout our lives, and walk back with us through it all to heal the wounds that have remained. Along with that healing, he longs to help us stand with him in forgiveness toward all those who have inflicted that pain. It has been my experience in co-laboring with Jesus for someone's healing, that once a person meets Jesus in their pain with his healing touch, forgiveness easily follows. Forgiveness never excuses or says the person wasn't wrong, it simply allows God to be their judge. It frees *us* to get on with our own lives.

CHAPTER 10

As we learn to cooperate with Jesus there, a new redemption begins to enter our lives that goes far beyond just going to heaven when we die – it is a redemption of pain. Unfortunately pain has been a part of all of our stories. When in an un-redeemed state it is destructive to ourselves and to others, and gives the enemy a victory. As we become willing to face our wounds and the painful emotions they caused us, meet Jesus in that place, and release to him the people that caused our pain through forgiving them, an exchange is made. We trade our hurts and wounds for his healing love and acceptance. *"Surely he took up our infirmities and carried our sorrows... by his wounds we are healed."* (Isaiah 53:4 & 5b) That is the redemption of what the enemy has tried to steal, kill, and destroy. (John 10:10)

I have had the joy of walking with countless people as they became willing to walk out of their woundedness onto the journey of fighting for the life that was robbed from them through the pain of living in this broken world. God hates the *robbery* that happened in the lives he paid for. So must we despise that robbery, because it keeps us trapped under the grip of the enemy and crippled. (Isaiah 61:8) Wounded people wound others. We have all hurt others without even meaning to. I recently learned of a way I had hurt someone close to me very unintentionally. It cut deeply to my core because my heart's desire is to be a life-giver and a restorer of broken hearts. I desire to co-labor with Jesus as a life-giver. However, sadly in that case, I did the opposite. When we see that we all hurt one another, even at times when we are totally unaware, living a lifestyle of forgiveness becomes essential. In these days, just about every time I see someone do something hurtful, the Spirit brings it right back to me and I begin to see how often I have done the same even without meaning to. We all come short of the way we were originally meant to be. (Romans 3:23)

When we are willing to cooperate with him, Jesus is able to begin the process of untangling the twisted mess that comes along with the lies the enemy has whispered to us through our pain. Then God's truth, light, life, and redemption is brought into those places. As healing begins to touch the depths of our beings, it affects us in other ways as well – in our physical health, our ways of relating, our motives for doing things, and the speech that comes out of a heart that is now being redeemed. When we refuse to forgive but remain resentful and bitter, the unforgiveness becomes like a toxin within us, poisoning ourselves and others. We learn from the book of Hebrews that when resentment and unforgiveness remain in our hearts, a root of bitterness then begins to grow up on the inside of us that brings defilement to many. (Hebrews 12:15)

Paul in speaking of the disputes that were going on involving the believers in 1 Corinthians 6, said, *"Do you not know that the saints will judge the world?"* Or in verse 3, *"Do you not know that we will judge angels?..."* Scripture after scripture points to a new heaven and a new earth in which we will have a meaningful part to play. In the meantime though, during this preparation period, we will continue to live with partial mystery, living by faith in a good God who will bring forth his good purposes. (Revelation 21 & 22)

The Fruit of Redemption

I just had someone tell me yesterday that as they glanced at themselves in the mirror, they realized they were now standing straighter! That new erectness came from a heart that is more and more living in redemption. As the pain we've experienced gets healed and redeemed, it makes a way for our redeemed pain to flow out from us to bring healing to others. Just as wounded people wound, healed people heal. We begin to join Jesus as ministers of reconciliation and redemption without even trying. What had been stolen and subtracted from us is now multiplied out to countless others with love. It's like throwing a pebble in a pond and watching

CHAPTER 10

the ripples go forth. We were just the pebble – we didn't try to make the ripples, they simply happened because we were willing to be dropped into the unknown waters of the pond. That is true in families as well, the ripples begin to touch our children in a new way that gives them hope and an example for redemption, even though they still must take their own journey.

The book of Hebrews reminds us that Jesus endured the cross and all its agony for the joy that was set beyond it – that joy was for us being freed for life eternal and to really become who we were always meant to be. It frees us to live and co-labor with him forever, fulfilling his ultimate purposes in this earth and beyond. Our purposes don't end when we die – this phase of our journey on earth is simply training for reigning even beyond our death. We need a larger perspective of life and eternity than many Christians currently have. How many Christians have secretly questioned that perhaps this life here is really all there is.

John the Baptist, even after he had heard the Father's audible voice and seen the Spirit descend on Jesus while baptizing him in the Jordan, questioned. It is human to question and even healthy – we need to allow our hearts to struggle through our fears and questions in order to apprehend these truths for ourselves. It takes our being willing to know and trust him in a way that allows us to be fully honest. When our former denial gets broken, usually through difficult circumstances, we are forced to begin to face the reality of the brokenness that is all around us in a way we might never have before. Allowing ourselves the struggle with our doubts and fears often becomes a necessary part of our coming to true faith that sustains.

In healing ministry, I have walked with countless men and women, who have been Christians for years, that finally recognized the need to struggle through their previously hidden anger toward God and his ways. However, when first asked if they might have anger toward God because he didn't seemingly come through for them in the way they thought he should have, any anger was vehemently denied! But as they began to recognize they truly did have buried anger, it also became apparent to many how that anger, and the accompanying lack of trust in God, was daily playing out in their lives through the need to control or escape through various addictions. By facing their anger, they were able to recognize the lies they were believing on a deep level of the heart and wrestle with them in order to come to the truth of God's word and a new simple, child-like trust in God.

Living with Peace

To live with peace in the reality of how broken this world really is, we must have a greater reality that remains steady even when everything around us is quaking. That reality is God, our Rock, who is in control and who is mighty in our midst. We must recognize that this world is not what we were originally made for (that was the perfection of the Garden), and thankfully one day we will live continually in the reality of what we were really created for. This is not the end of our story, but only the training ground for the fullness of eternal purpose when Jesus fully completes the restoration process. One day we will experience the feast we are hungry for and live the life we were created for. All the growth that we allow here is a part of that – it doesn't end. One day our joy will be constant, our tears and sorrows completely washed away. One day we will be fully free to love and be loved the way we have always desired and have only had a taste of here. (Revelation 7:17 & 21:22-27)

(Hebrews 11:8-16) In these verses we find many of God's faithful ones still living by faith when they died even though there were promises that were only partially experienced. Verse 10 reminds us that (Abraham) *"was looking forward to the city with foundations, whose architect and builder is God."*

CHAPTER 10

Verse 13: *"All these people were still living by faith when they died. They did not receive the things promised; they only saw them and welcomed them from a distance. And they admitted that they were aliens and strangers on earth."*... (Verse 16) *"Instead, they were longing for a better country, a heavenly one. Therefore God is not ashamed to be called their God, for he has prepared a city for them."* And he has prepared a city for *us* as well where we will at last be completely fulfilled.

In the meantime, how do we handle the ache within our hearts since we were made for so much more, for the perfection of the Garden? We groan. Romans 8 speaks of both the suffering now and the future glory we will partake of later. Verse 18, *"I consider that our present sufferings are not worth comparing with the glory that will be revealed in us. The creation waits in eager expectation for the sons of God to be revealed."* In the meantime, our internal groaning is natural as we wait for the fulfillment of all we were created for. *"We know that the whole creation has been groaning as in the pains of childbirth right up to the present time. Not only so, but we ourselves, who have the first fruits of the Spirit, groan inwardly as we wait eagerly for our adoption as sons, the redemption of our bodies."* (Romans 8:22-23) 1 Corinthians 15:35 to the end gives us a further glimpse of our resurrection bodies.

We can't honestly face the reality of the world we are currently living in as it is without groaning. Groaning can sometimes feel like a bad thing, but it's actually not. When we face reality as it is, we are living in truth, and so we are set free. If you are honest, can't you feel the groaning? I can. Could that be what we have been trying to cover over with busyness and addictions of all kinds? (Even the good ones like Bible knowledge, helping people, etc.)? These might include seeking sensual pleasures of all kinds, unhealthy relationships, successes, and on and on?

There is an empty place within us all that will never be fully filled until we are released from this body to live in the world for which we were created. However in the meantime, as we discover our true selves, even while experiencing the groaning now, we can enter the eternal joy of co-laboring with Jesus. God can pour water on our thirsty souls, and we can experience his tremendous love and acceptance right where we are. And from that place of cooperation with him in his purposes, we have the amazing opportunity to bear fruit that lasts for all of eternity! Fruit that remains!

In 2 Corinthians 5:1-10, Paul speaks of our groaning. *"Now we know that if the earthly tent we live in is destroyed, we have a building from God, an eternal house in heaven, not built by human hands. Meanwhile we groan, longing to be clothed with our heavenly dwelling, because when we are clothed, we will not be found naked. For while we are in this tent, we groan and are burdened..."*

"We know that the whole creation has been groaning as in the pains of childbirth right up to the present time. Not only so, but we ourselves, who have the first fruits of the Spirit, groan inwardly as we wait eagerly for our adoption as sons, the redemption of our bodies." (Romans 8:22-23)

Coming to Terms with Death as a Part of Life

1 Thessalonians 4:13, *"Brothers, we do not want you... to grieve like the rest of men who have no hope."*

As we walk with God through our own personal wilderness season, we do often grieve for what we had hoped our lives would have looked like. In that season, nothing seems to work and we can feel thwarted on every side. We grieve the false hopes we didn't even realize we had. They get exposed as we journey the rough terrain in that particular season.

CHAPTER 10

Prior to our wilderness season, we have often lived with many hopes – for example, we have hoped life would turn out a certain way, that our spouse would change, we hoped for a friend or loved one to be healed of cancer, we hoped our kids would stop running from the Lord, we hoped our finances would have quickly turned around, and on and on. When heaven seems silent and those hopes are first thwarted, our hearts tend to become sick (Proverbs 13:12) and we often begin to experience despair and hopelessness on a deeper level than perhaps we have known before. That often happens when there are many dashed hopes all piling up at once.

The disciples experienced that loss of hope on the Road to Emmaus in Luke 24:21. They had a certain picture of how Jesus would save the world, and when he died, their hopes were smashed. That same thing happens to us when we have a certain picture of how something should be. The phrase in that Scripture that will forever stick in my mind is a very painful one we have all experienced over and over... *"but we had hoped..."*. Jesus then revealed himself to them in the breaking of the bread and re-interpreted the scriptures to them.

When our hopes are disappointed, a fear of despair can then begin to raise its ugly head. But we should have a fear of despair, right? Of course we know that despair can go into a dark place, as we have witnessed far too many times in people who have fallen into deep depressions, suicides, etc., but despair is meant to be a *"door of hope"*. In Hosea 2:15 we see the Valley of Trouble (Achor) becoming a *door of hope*. It is sometimes not until despair hits us that our other false hopes begin to get broken because we can no longer make our desires happen no matter how much we try to control or pray. Amazingly, through the despair something new begins to happen... through facing that despair a new hope in God is quietly birthed. This hope is not one that any longer requires God to do things a certain way. Out of our previous hopelessness a new hope begins to arise, but this hope is in God alone and it's the beginning of a belief that we truly will see *"the goodness of God in the land of the living"*, no matter what that happens to look like. (Psalm 27:13,14)

When we are willing to "die" to our former more shallow hopes, a new resurrection life begins to come forth through us. We begin to see larger than we previously had and realize more clearly that this life is not really all about us. Instead, the life we then live begins to become more about God and our working with him to fulfill the purposes he ordained for us from before we were ever born. Our life begins to take on more of an eternal quality as we simply remain present each day – no longer living for whatever success or pleasure we can manage to eek out of it, but instead, joining him in fulfilling his kingdom purposes. We begin to see larger than we ever have before and how our particular story fits into his. We begin to enter into the mysteries of God, and even though we can still only see through a glass partially, our hearts become more awakened than ever before. *"Arise, shine, for your light has come, and the glory of the Lord rises upon you. See, darkness covers the earth and thick darkness is over the peoples, but the Lord rises upon you and his glory appears over you."* (Isaiah 60:1,2)

"Loving Not Their Lives Unto Death" (Revelation 12:11)

Death is too often a taboo subject. Frequently, as Christians, we tend to avoid talking about it even when a friend or loved one is dying. As a result, they are forced to struggle through, feeling isolated and alone. In fact, sometimes in our well-meaning attempts to help, and certainly without realizing it, we too often either get preachy or very subtly put guilt on them that they don't have enough faith for healing. That can be so painful for someone who is already struggling.

CHAPTER 10

That faithful man of God, Judson Cornwall, in the midst of the journey toward his own death, writes in his last book, <u>Dying With Grace</u>, *"There is something about suffering most of us Christians don't understand. We see the dealings of God as being very temporal and that it is his blessed will to heal everyone. Yet the Bible speaks of fulfilling the sufferings of Christ. I am not sure we understand that very well. We feel there should be no suffering or pain, yet all through the Scriptures we see chosen ones of God enduring suffering and pain."*

We do need to pray for healing – the scripture tells us so. But first, do we need to seek God to see if this is their time to go Home to be with Him? Is this a time when their season on earth might be finished? Have they finished their particular race? Have they completed what God had prepared for them before they were ever born? (Ps. 139:13-16) If we hear that this is their time, we will be praying with Jesus the great intercessor himself, and pray according to the will of God. If after asking him, we are still not clear, how wonderful it is to be able to pray in the Spirit. The scripture in Romans 8:26-27 reminds us that, *"the Spirit helps in our weakness. We do not know what we ought to pray for, but the Spirit himself intercedes for us with groans that words cannot express. And he who searches our hearts knows the mind of the Spirit, because the Spirit intercedes for the saints in accordance with God's will."*

As I shared earlier, I felt God lovingly prepared me much earlier in the year that my husband would die before the year's end. As it turned out, Bruce passed over on December 29th, but until just a very short time before his death, hours in fact, it did not appear that way. I was sure I had heard wrongly, and even when he was in the hospital the week prior to his death, the doctors were declaring he would recover from this latest episode. Yet all the while they were saying that, I felt in my heart that this was the end of his journey. Some time after his passing, the Lord spoke to me that Bruce had gone as far as he could go and that God was pleased. He had finished his race.

I desire my life to be used for God's purposes. Although I do not want to go home one day early until I have completed what I have been placed on this earth to do. I also do not want to remain one day beyond my ordained time to cross over. Although I can't say I understand all of this, I do not want even the earnest, heart-felt prayers of well-meaning loved ones to keep me here beyond my time. For years, I have pondered the scriptures of Hezekiah's illness and healing in Isaiah chapters 38 & 39. The Lord clearly revealed to Hezekiah to put his house in order because he would not recover from his illness, however because of Hezekiah's agonizing prayer, The Lord gave him fifteen more years. That all sounds good, except that little did Hezekiah know, in the fifteen years after his healing, trouble would come. As we read in 2 Kings 20:18, *"And some of your descendants, your own flesh and blood, that will be born to you, will be taken away, and they will become eunuchs in the palace of the King of Babylon."* I have also pondered Isaiah 57:1, *"The righteous perish, and no one ponders it in his heart; devout men are taken away, and no one understands that the righteous are taken away to be spared of evil."*

A friend whose time was approaching to leave this earth and be present with the Lord wrote me a sad letter. Well meaning loved ones and friends would not release her and would not allow her to speak about dying. She desired to share what God had been showing her in her heart that her time on this earth was finished. As a result, until I wrote to her and shared with her about the new journey she was about to embark on, there was no one she could really talk with about it. Because of my letter, she called me and we spoke about the one thing dearest to her heart at that point in her life, her passing from this earth to her real Home. She could speak about the excitement of finally seeing Jesus face to face and seeing her three beloved children who had gone on before.

CHAPTER 10

Instead of a time of joyful sharing with many around her, she was forced to pass over with just a few who understood. What a wonderful time of deep heart-sharing death can be if we can truly enter in with someone whose time on this earth is ending – sorrowful yes, but joyful as well.

We can be a part of the death of those we care about as well as a part of their life. It saddens me to know that I have not always been emotionally present in the way I handled the passing over of certain loved ones. I wish I had a do-over, but unfortunately life doesn't always give us that so the most I could do was to ask Jesus to let them know how sorry I was. It is so easy to shut down emotionally and just do the many tasks at hand at a time like that, or to be there in body, but disconnected from the struggles of the heart. Just as we desire to be emotionally present in the happy celebrations of a loved-one's life, so must we be present with them in the sorrowful as well.

Another special friend who was deeply mourning the loss of her teenage daughter who went Home seemingly far too early, said that the gift of salvation meant more to her than ever before because it promised my friend that one day she would have a joyful reunion with her daughter! Therefore, in the midst of her horrendous grief, because of the cross, she had hope.

Are there days coming somewhere down the road when there will be great loss of life on this earth? The book of Revelation tells us that is so. We do not know when, but could God be desiring to prepare us to die as well as to live? Could it be that even if what is described in the book of Revelation is not in our lifetime, is it possible that we are not really free until we are able to die as well as live? Does our fear of death give the enemy an open door to torment? Jesus said he overcame that fear for us. *"...by his death he might destroy him who holds the power of death – that is, the devil and free those who all their lives were held in slavery by their fear of death."* (Hebrews 2:14-15). *"They overcame him (Satan) by the blood of the Lamb and by the word of their testimony; they did not love their lives so much as to shrink from death."* (Rev. 12:11)

As Christians, have we somehow bought into the world's way of viewing death? Have we shared in their *"legitimate fear of death"*? For without a Savior, death should be rightfully feared. Jesus took the sting out of death, making it now just a changing of locations. When my husband Bruce died, I kept thinking that now he was just living in a different country from me. It was almost like he was living in India or someplace – I had never yet been there personally even though I had read about it. One day I would travel there too, but for now he was just on the other side of the veil. One day, probably in the not too distant future, I will be joining him in that country.

Have we endeavored to make this earth our "heaven"? (Hebrews 11:13-16), vs. 16 says, *"Instead they were longing for a better country – a heavenly one. Therefore God is not ashamed to be called their God, for he has prepared a city for them."* As Christians we know that our lives don't end at death, but do we sometimes live that way? The reality is that through death, we will be enjoying a whole new dimension of freedom that will enable us to more fully fulfill the purposes of our existence. In the book, Dying with Grace by Judson Cornwall, states, *"Those who have died in Christ have not been cheated out of life; they have been metamorphosed into the real life."* Then he states, *"The beauties of heaven and unhindered life with God Himself defy our imagination."* We can't begin to picture it all because we really have no paradigm for anything that perfect.

Do we need to more fully embrace an eternal viewpoint of life? Have we somehow missed the truth that for a Christian, death is just an event (like many of the other events we experience) on the journey of life? *"I eagerly expect and hope*

CHAPTER 10

that I will in no way be ashamed, but will have sufficient courage so that now as always Christ will be exalted in my body, whether by life or by death. For to me, to live is Christ and to die is gain." (Philippians 1:20-21)

To truly prepare us for the life God has for us, do we need to rethink what we believe about death? Why do so many Christians fight so hard to live when they are dying? Do we unconsciously see our life as we know it, as the end? It is one thing if we sense our purposes on this earth have not yet been finished and it is the enemy who is trying to steal, kill, and destroy, but have we heard that from God? I don't believe we always know if our purpose has been completed or not. If we believe that we are to hold onto this life at all costs, we cannot accept that death is another valid experience on our journey of life. Death is a part of life to the Christian! Paul spoke that absence from the body is presence with the Lord. Perhaps we must rethink our view of "eternal life"? Do we just see it as something that happens when we die? For someone with a relationship with Jesus, we are already living in eternal life!

Jesus said in John 17:3 *"Now this is eternal life; that they may know You, the only true God and Jesus Christ, whom you have sent."* If we have received Jesus, and if we are moving more and more toward intimacy with him, then to pass over through death is simply to at last know him face to face and to be able to finally fully become like him. Since we first received Jesus into our lives, we have been moving toward that fullness of discovery. Isn't becoming like Jesus our desire even now? Death in Jesus, and in his timing, is a culmination of all that our hearts have longed for. It is an exciting adventure and simply a journey with Jesus in crossing over into an undiscovered country. *"...we shall be like Him for we shall see Him as He is."* (1 John 3:2b)

These are hard questions that we need to wrestle through with God. How does he view death? That is a question for each of us to ask him to reveal to us personally. I share these things that I have struggled through to a place of peace, to provoke you to seek God's truth for yourself. Someone I know who recently passed over, even though a Christian for many, many years, sadly struggled in the days prior to his death because he had never wrestled this through for himself earlier.

"Precious in the sight of the Lord is the death of His saints." (Psalm 116:15)

"For to me, to live is Christ and to die is gain." (Philippians 2:21)

"For I am convinced that neither death nor life, neither angels nor demons, neither the present nor the future, nor any powers, neither height nor depth, nor anything else in all creation, will be able to separate us from the love of God that is in Christ Jesus our Lord." (Romans 8:38-39)

We have much to look ahead to, but at the same time, so much co-laboring with Jesus in our own unique way *today!* Our lives are needed! You are on this earth for *such a time as this.*

The End of the Story

The new heaven and the new earth: (Revelation 21 & 22) (Isaiah 66:22-24)

"Then I saw a new heaven and a new earth, for the first heaven and the first earth had passed away, and there was no longer any sea. I saw the Holy City, the new Jerusalem, coming down out of heaven from God, prepared as a bride beautifully dressed for her husband. And I heard a loud voice from the throne saying, 'Now the dwelling of God is with men, and he will live with them. They will be his people, and God himself

CHAPTER 10

will be with them and be their God. He will wipe every tear from their eyes. There will be no more death or mourning or crying or pain, for the old order of things has passed away'. He who was seated on the throne said, 'I am making everything new!' Then he said, 'Write this down, for these words are trustworthy and true.'" (Revelation 21:1-5)

One day we will finally taste all we were created to experience if we had been able to remain in the Garden. The deepest desires of our hearts will be filled to overflowing. How exciting it will be to have the opportunity to participate with him in the new heaven and new earth! For now, if we will continue to surrender our wills to his, and allow him to mold us into the fullness of our original design – we will one day experience an amazing adventure of co-labor with Jesus on that new earth. At long last, there will be no more darkness or groaning, sickness or sorrow, but fullness of joy without measure! Whatever training and preparation we are currently going through will all be worth it for we will reign with Jesus in his glory!

"...No eye has seen, no ear has heard, no mind has conceived what God has prepared for those who love him." (1 Corinthians 2:9

A PARTIAL EMOTIONS LIST

Categories of Emotions and Some of the Subtle Ways They Can Be Experienced

HURT: Feeling wounded, distressed, offended, injured, abused, used, harmed, pained, sorrowful, suffering, grieved, sad, brokenhearted, disappointed, discouraged, rejected, abandoned, shamed

FEAR: Feeling anxious, panic, terror, apprehension, alarm, afraid, suspicious, distrusting, worried, over-concerned, troubled, uneasy, anguished, agitated, disquieted, unbelieving

ANGER: Feeling rage-full, aggressive, depressed (anger turned inward), rebellious, resentful, bitter, desire to punish, frustrated, contemptuous, disrespectful, hostile, annoyed, furious, argumentative, combative, sulky, irritated, outraged, arrogant, antagonizing, overwhelmed, misunderstood, unappreciated, powerless (can fuel anger), having inward or outward tantrums

GUILT (REAL OR FALSE): Feeling judgmental, critical, envious, always feeling guilty, wanting to hide, self-condemning, disgraceful, disconnected, powerless, isolated, self-condemning

SHAME (REAL OR FALSE): Feeling insignificant, worthless, a failure, unworthy, embarrassed, unimportant, unwanted, useless, self-sabotaging, forgotten, forsaken, inadequate, insecure, not valuable, discarded, unneeded, disgraceful, self-depreciating, invisible, wanting to hide behind a false self (wearing a mask)

GRIEF: Feeling sad, sorrowful, undone, distracted, withdrawn, angry, tearful, brokenhearted, overwhelmed

A false shame belief can reveal itself as pride by feeling *"more than others"*. (Romans 12:3)

ASK GOD TO REVEAL:

I am angry because_____

I feel fear of _____ because_____

Is my guilt real or false?_____

I feel shame about who I am because _____

Is my shame driving me to pride?_____

When negative emotions are owned and processed, they can release positive emotions.

EXAMPLES:
- Anger and fear when faced and released can become courage

- Fear when heart-surrendered to God becomes peace

- Real guilt & shame when acknowledged and forgiven enables us to experience forgiveness, rest, and peace

- False shame when released can bring truth into our innermost being and give us a healthy self image that comes from the life of Jesus within us (Colossians 1:27)

COURAGE: Can be experienced as repentance, boldness, the ability to experience God's delegated authority, bravery, passion, perseverance, persistence, the ability to wait, strength

PEACE: Can be experienced as becoming more trusting, drawing life out of God's wisdom, feeling restful, more secure, relaxed, confident, joyous, light-hearted, carefree, having increased Godly dependency

FORGIVENESS: Can be experienced as feeling accepted, secure, belonging, loved, having approval, feeling cared for, at peace and at rest, and helps us to develop a thankful heart

GRIEF: When mourned through can bring us to acceptance and the ability to move on (even while still recognizing and honoring the loss) into a new season of life. Joy can then be released through facing our sorrows.

Our emotions are the voice of our hearts and when they have been denied and pushed down, we lose our true selves. We can then begin to live out of an image or behind a mask. We then *"do" (a human doing) instead of "be" (a human being).*

THE RESULT: Burnout, dullness, drudgery, boredom, joylessness, problems with intimacy, unable to have deep heart-connections with God or people.

Jesus came to heal the broken-hearted. (Isaiah 61:1)

REFERENCES

Oswald Chambers. *My Utmost for His Highest*

Pat Stark. *Born to Fly*

Dr. Henry Cloud & Dr. John Towsend. *Boundaries*

Mrs. Charles E. Cowman. *Streams in the Desert*

Judson Cornwall. *Dying with Grace*

Sarah Young, *Jesus Calling*

All Scriptures, unless otherwise indicated, are taken from the Holy Bible, New International Version.

Pursuing the life you were meant to live... *free*

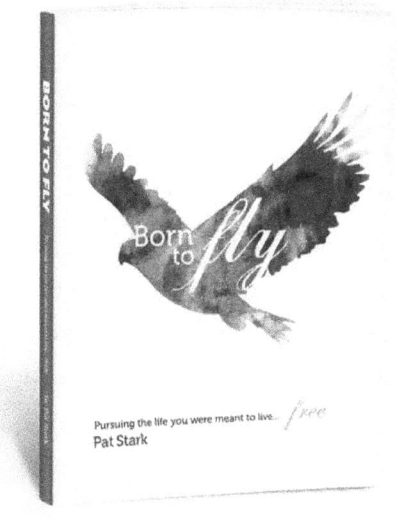

- Are you desiring freedom, peace, and healing in your life?
- Are you weary of feeling trapped in the mundane struggles of life?
- Are you searching for the way to spiritual and emotional healing and restoration?
- Are you desiring to discover who you really are and who you were originally created to be?

Born to Fly
by Pat Stark

Find the keys that can enable you to cooperate with the Holy Spirit in becoming free from bondages of the past, thereby releasing you to live more fully in the present with excitement toward your future.

Available for purchase at www.Amazon.com and www.thecovenantcenter.com/store
$12.99 Paperback / $6.99 Kindle

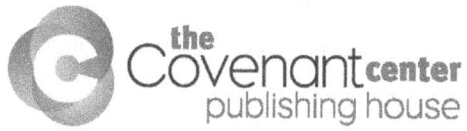

TESTIMONIALS FOR
BORN TO FLY, by Pat Stark

"As you read this book and begin to allow God to walk you through your own healing journey, I pray that even if you never have the joy of knowing Pat personally the gift God has put in her to counsel, guide, encourage, admonish and fight for others would be as real and present for you as it has been for me. And I encourage you to keep going. Don't give up! Keep this process as a priority for your life because in the end you will find the result of God's transformation - a life that is new, real, strange and wonderful. He is faithful and I continue to pray 'God, don't leave me in my condition.'"

~Heather

"Your book is speaking to me right where I am. So loudly, in fact, that when I did as you suggested and read the Table of Contents to see which chapters spoke to me, I found that I had highlighted ALL of them! :) I also have highlighted so much that it's a majority of each page. :)"

~Christina

"What a life-changing gift it has been for me to begin to work through this process of rediscovering my own heart. Meeting and getting to know the little girl in my childhood pictures has given me back my life. For a long time, I struggled with loneliness, depression, and a poor self-image. I felt 'stuck' and just couldn't seem to ever 'get on with things'. I was living with so much disappointment and so many unfulfilled longings and didn't know how to even begin to change that. Committing myself to the process of pursuing my heart has brought incredible healing to my brokenness, and it has without a doubt been key to getting 'unstuck'. My life felt like a movie on 'pause', but something about this process has pushed 'play' *(wow!!)... Now as I have been learning to see, value, love, and live fully from my own heart (instead of living behind a mask) – in the present – being ok with myself and all of my 'messiness', I am actually enjoying myself, and loving my life!"*

~Chalis

"For many years, I lived like a chicken scratching in the scorched soil searching for sustenance. After reading and re-reading, <u>Born to Fly</u>, God's truths are replacing my false beliefs. Pat shares straight from her heart: we are created to soar as eagles secure in Holy Spirit's strength rather than striving on our own. His truth sets us free indeed to be who He made us to be! Pat's practical and encouraging nuggets of Scriptural wisdom are born from experience; she challenges me to change!"

~Beth

"I think today was the first day in my life that I actually started liking myself. I know that may sound weird, but I have been in so much self condemnation about my past failures and inability to 'live a normal life' and all my fears. I blamed myself all along. It is staggering to realize my fear of failure, my procrastination in life, my fear of being rejected all stems from my fear of being shamed. This was not my fault. This was something that happened to me. I was unable and incapable of protecting myself from this damage. It was not my fault, period. And I blamed myself all these years, every day of my life, without even knowing it."

~Eileen

"Been reading your book and the timing is just right. My childhood past is being restored through the Spirit of The Lord and your book."

~Frank

"It was a great breakthrough reading Pat's first book. Instead of using self-protection I was able to face my deep emotions, grieve the pain and loss and walk into healing, with no strings attached."

~ Nancy

"I just could not get over the vision I got of that poor little girl (me) being swept up into Jesus' arms, and the little girl just screaming at the top of her lungs and trying to squeeze herself out of Jesus' arms, because she was so absolutely terrified. That was me. That is me. It is no wonder I have been so bound up all my life! In the vision, Jesus did not let her go, and held on tight to her."

~Another Testimony

www.ingramcontent.com/pod-product-compliance
Lightning Source LLC
Chambersburg PA
CBHW060526100426
42743CB00009B/1442